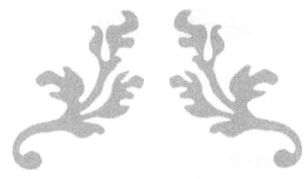

CURE

FARUK BURAK

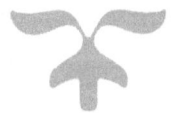

CURE

Your eyes told to me
When you are gone
After those fancy words..
The sound of footsteps coming up the stairs..
Pressed to my head to my head,
Your ran from the facts
When you go downhill
You thought it would be better,
Fire of love pressed onto your skin
Temperature of my skin
Flowed from your nape
My kisses poured to ground
From your lips,
As long as you continue to walk
My eyes stuck to your thoughts,
Now how you will take a breath?
Goodbye.
'Faruk BURAK'

SYMPTOM

Winter was about to be over, Fikret began to wait in front of the statue of Ulus Square to go to the Museum of Anatolian Civilizations. The sun began to lightly lighten the bones, but the wind was still cold. There was not much to see, there were no women in the square, and the looks of those around did not look good either. They seemed like a tribe out of sight. The people who looked like soldiers, whorebreakers, swindlers and murderers on the weekend, ready to attack at any moment, waiting quietly in the corner, and unknown where they came from. Five minutes had passed and Ali had not come yet.

Fikret:

-Alo, where are you Ali? Are you coming from Fizan?

Ali:

- Fikret i m on my way, I'm in the center of the Red Crescent.

Fikret:

-You said you'd meet me at half-past.I think you went out in the middle of the noon.

Ali:

-I will be there soon ,sorry..

Fikret:

- Will it take five minutes?

Ali:

- I believe that's the most..

Fikret:

-Anyway ... I'm waiting for ...

Fikret, decided to move around as far as the Ali.. It was very remarkable to wait in the same spot for a long time and the clothes on it could make itself a target and did not want to encounter a problem while standing still.He startes to headway. First, he mixed up with people gathered to watch the show who selling medicinal herbs .. But the man tells of - Adam Otu - did not take much interest and went on. A little farther, those on the pavement near the entrance of a building looked out and approached. Five elderly men had formed a circle. The oldest one were sitting and there was a simple table in front of him, He quickly mixed the three cards of his hand, put it in front of his other friends and he said that he will pay twice as much money as who puts on joker. Fikret came a little closer to see what was going on and started watching. To the right of the sitting man, a tall man was watching around and game. It seemed like he was controlling. There was an old man who seemed to play right in front of him. The old man was mixes the cards and set out him in front of him,then He was called -Bul Karayı Al Parayı-.The old man was constantly losing. Fikret was watching the man's hand movements very carefully and could see what the dark was. But he did not take much time to realize there was a serious trickery. There were two other people to the right and left of the old man playing the game and someone was talking constantly and very fast. Approached to Fikret:

Man:

-Look at the man who is constantly losing very pity, Let's curl the corner of the paper and make some money for the guy..Well?

-Let show...

But the old man still continued to lose. Fikret was even more certain that these five people knew each other very well. The man who broke the corner of the paper stopped and stood still:

Man:

- I'm playing these two hundred liras for this young friend, then he put the money on a piece of paper.

- You won!Take your Money..Lets go!

Fikret:

-No ..No.Noo..Thanks..

On a sudden everyone started to break up. Fikret was not surprised and understood that they were trying to pull him into the game. The men were very surprised that Fikret did not get the money. But Fikret did not tell the man to play at my place, nor gave money. All of the people knew each other and set up the trickery.. Fikret did not have such a plot. It did not take much time to understand that the money in his hand was fake. It was very easy to break the plans of the people by laughing sincerely.

Man:

- Thank you, brother.

- Take your Money..

Fikret:

- Come on, thank you ..

Said and he continued to walk upwards. Before too late he came back to the square and saw that Ali was looking for him around.

Fikret:

-Ali ... Ali ..

-My friend..How you do?

Ali:

-I'm fine ..

Fikret:
- Let's just get out of here.
-I do not think anyone should wait here for more than fifteen minutes.

Ali:
-I'm sorry, Fikret.

Fikret:
-Anyway, no problem ... Let's look at our work.
-Look at the pile of slum that is in the middle of the city. How ugly looks ..

Ali:
-Actually this area has been completely emptied and I still do not know why it has not demolished. It looks disgusting, does not it?

Fikret:
-Yes, my friend, I think they need to clean this place right away.

Fikret and Ali, talk while walking, realized that they had come to the front of the museum.

Ali:
-Do you have a bank credit card, Fikret?

Fikret:
-Where ... I do not use credit cards.

Ali:
- I can get a discount.

Fikret:
- No bro.

Ali:
- OK..

Fikret:

-Ali here as much as the back garden of the Istanbul Archaeological Museum.

-There's something really crazy.

Ali:
- OK..

Fikret:
- Look at the skull. How many years ago?

Ali:
-B.C. 2800 Fikret ..

Fikret:
-No monkey is like a skull.

Ali:
-You are crazy Fikret .

Fikret:
-Bro I say, this Darwin raised his head in time, looked at the people around him, and when he saw that they really lived like monkeys, he told them they came from the monkeys, and he convinced them to that, and the good wave went well.

-Did he write his theory in Oxford?

Ali:
-Yeah, Ali ...hahaha..

Fikret:

-When we looked at the arts and technology of this Hittite civilization, the symbols used in the religious ceremonies of many of the works were very prominent. Especially these swastikas were attracted to my attention...

Ali:

-They used it, did not they, Fikret?

Fikret:

-Yes..This pagan believes that swastika is towards the right represents goodness and the if it is towards the left represents evil ..

Ali:

- These are to the left.

Fikret:

-Yeah, but look at this one, as one of the crucifix symbols used in Christianity right now. I started to believe that the Christian world had carried many pagan beliefs and symbols into this religion and maintained this belief in the same way.

-These are ... well, there are some kind of cross symbols in Christianity.

-Maybe these signs reinforce our scheme.

- The sun, the cross and the swastika.

-I think that religious beliefs have spread to the world at that time and formed a culture because we can encounter the same symbolic signs and works of art in many parts of the world .. I believe that this is still going on ..

Ali:

-You maybe right..I came here with a lot of people. But you're making the most interesting comments. Look this part is from the time of King Midas.

Fikret:

-Mmm.Frigya..that they were united with the Urartu and fought against the Assyrians?

Ali:

- Yes, my friend.

Fikret:

-I think Midas, Hittites did not deal with religion works like a lot .. Simple and far away from religion artworks are striking ..

Ali:

- I guess so...

Fikret:

-If only this museum was my house ... would it be crazy?

Ali:

-Way, it's different.

Fikret:

-If not as much as Midas, I was live here like a king.

Ali:

-Did you like it ?

Fikret:

-I liked ..Thank you for this activity.

Ali:

-You're welcome..

Fikret:

-Although it is not a very big museum, it is was good that we come here today.

Ali:

-Yeah, I think so too...

-What do we do now, Fikret?

Fikret:

-I do not know..

Ali:

-I know a nice café right there, we can drink Turkish coffee inside, what do you say?

Fikret:

-Ok .. I m tired ..It will be good..

Ali:

-Let's get out of here.

Fikret and Ali had a long and steep slope and then they came to the entrance of the café .. They opened the door and they went inside.Inside smelled of pasta and garlic.They sat down on a floor, one of the tables that saw the view of Ankara in the distance.

Waiter:

-You're welcome, sir.

Ali:

- Do you have hot cocoa?

Waiter:

- No, not..

Ali:

- Do you have Turkish coffee?

Waiter:

- No.

Ali:

- What do you have? ... Is there tea?

Waiter:

-There is..

Ali:

-2 tea please.

Fikret:

- Ali, this swastika thing is very interesting today. I want to tell you a theory.

Ali:

-Ok..

Fikret:

- Here's a map of the world. Here's the Middle East, this is Europe, this is the Americas, and Australia is the next. These include the Atlantic Ocean and the Pacific Ocean.

Ali:

-Yeah..

Fikret:

- I think before the Noah's Flood there are major landmasses in this Atlantic Ocean and the Pacific Ocean. I think Atlantis is above Atlantic Ocean and Lemuria is Pacific.I say to MU part of from Afghanistan's capital Kabul to Japan ..

Ali:

- Yea..

Fikret:

- Now, when God fired Satan, he sent the devil and his folk to Lemuria. Adam came to the sides of southern Arabia. Adam and Eve met here. Then their children were Kabul with Abel.

Ali:

-Yeah..

Fikret:

- Now tell me ... Where is the capital city of Afghanistan?

Ali:

-Kabul..

Fikret:

-Well, then, Kabul became a descendant here, and the descendants of the devil and the descendants of the Kabul came into contact with each other and began to contact with each other. Satan began to teach people many things that should not be taught. They started to have sexual relations with the descendants of the human race and the descendants of the devil. These sexual relations have begun to be children of another kind. As some of these children are very short and small, some of them have turned into great giants and spread to the world. This new race and these racial races , With the teachings of the devils to them, and perhaps even advanced than today's technology.I think so their beliefs were more like worshiping Satan.

-I think that today's religions are also based on this ..
Ali:
-Yeah..
Fikret:
- Can I have an ashtray?
Waiter:
-I'm sorry, sir.
Fikret:
- God was very angry and angry with this situation.
After that, huge giant race started to attack everything around this and started destroying everything. At that time God sent Noah as a prophet. He wanted to warn the people of this world.

-But Noah's prophet prayed and saved the world from a doom. He talked about a great flood to his people.
- This flood was really like a doom. Well, in this flood, Atlantis and Lemuria , was shattered with huge rocks descending from the skies and buried under the waters, ending a great world civilization.
Ali:
- Yeah..
-The next time, Noah's ship sat in a place and a new beginning for the world began.
Ali:
-Yeah.

Fikret:

- Do you know about Zulkerney?

Ali:

-Yeah..

Fikret:

-After the flood, Zulkarneyn is going to control both the west and the east of the world. I think it is the most northerly western part of Japan and England.

Ali:

-It's a theory.

Fikret:

-Yeah, this is my theory. I've done some research on this.

Remember that Zulkarneyn set aside a set of people on a mountain to cover underground.

-I think that the people who are trapped in the mountain are the giants of this demon and human race and the small short breed.

Ali:

-I do not agree with that.

Fikret:

-Why?

Ali:

-It will not affect my life if they have their presence or not.

Fikret:

- I do not understand .. What do you mean?

Ali:

-I cannot comprehend such things because of that, I do not say anything ... How do you know they will land from a hill?

Fikret:

-Take a look at the sura of the Kahf ... The Gog and Magog will flow from every hill

Ali:

-Yes i looked now ... I'm sure you're right ...

Ali had not really fully understood what Fikret was telling, and he did not have much information on it. He had heard it was ridiculous to say something, not to look like he did not know.

Ali:

-Yes Fikret like you said in the book.. I cannot comprehend..Its like a dream..

Fikret:

-We do not even know the existence of Allah .It's too like a dream yeah?

Ali:

-Hmm..Must be sure that the creator of this world.

Fikret:

-I do not have doubts, Ali.

-I've done a little research on my own.

Fikret and Ali were just drinking tea and the waiters were not happy at all. They came to the table and looked at the table and pressed to order something. Fikret was very uncomfortable about this and he hated these kinds of businesses. He always liked the cafes that noone came and stood up and waited for orders.

Ali:

-Dude, get up, let's go from this place.

Fikret:

-Let's go ... me too bothered ...

They gathered their goods over the table and left to go home. Ali had been a little sick because he talked to Fikret about the things he could not comment on, but it did not mean that these friendships would end. They left to go to their homes.

Fikret was going to return home to Istanbul in the night of that day. Every weekend he came to Ankara to visit his family. He was looking for his childhood friends whom he missed to spend the time. After this week, he spent a lot of time.After returning home and preparing his suitcase, he said good-bye to his family,and get on the Istanbul bus.He had just left the job and still could not find a new job. Time was working against him, he must supposed to be able to afford his house and all his expenses. Or he could have had to leave the city for nothing. He took a sleeping pill out of his pocket and rolled it to the tum. When Fikret was falling into the rush, the journey flowed like water. He put his backpack on his back and walked to the taxi stand at the entrance of the bus station.

Fikret:

-Good Morning..

Taxi Driver:

-Good morning... Where do you want to go?

Fikret:

- To Nishantasi ...

When Taxi entered Husrev Gerede Street, Fikret went down, walked for two or three minutes, then opened the house lock, threw the goods on the saloon, and laid on the sofa. All the lights were turned off, millions of thoughts flowed fast. He felt very thirsty, wanted to get up and drink, but never had to get up to his feet in his life. He had straightened his belly, then he slowly stood on his feet. The heart began to strike very fast,he was very sweaty and his left side was numb till his palms.

Fikret:

-I believe, I'm dying!

-What's happening to me?

-Do I have a heart attack? My God!

He slowly walked towards the kitchen, filled a glass of water, but he could only have a sip. He hugged his phone and immediately called a taxi, and he could barely barely find himself in the street. He started to wait taxi as stacked on the stairs in front of the apartment entrance. It was too late and he couldn't think call for anyone. Before long, the taxi came to the front of the door. The taxi driver who saw Fikret in that way came to his side and, after entering his arms, Fikret sat in the back seat.

Taxi Driver:

-Are you ok?

Fikret:

-No, I feel so bad, I think I'm having a heart attack, I can die right here.

-Please take me to the American Hospital immediately.

Taxi Driver:

- OK, calm down, I'll get you to the hospital as soon as possible.

Fikret:

- OK, quick, please ...

The taxi driver brought Fikret to the hospital and delivered it to the Emergency in a very short time.

Doctor:

-What do you have, sir?

Fikret:

-I feel so bad, I feel like my heart is squeezing, I can not breathe, my left colum is numb. My throat is dry..

Doctor:

- OK, sir, just stand here like this please.

Fikret had the first panic attack episode, and he did not realize it. The nurse after finding a vein in the his arm, The needle on the end of the serum was inserted into the his arm and Diazem started to fickle into the blood of Fikret ..

Fikret:

- Give me my phone, I want to call my family.

-Where's my phone?

Doctor:

- Here.

Fikret:

-Doctor, what do I have?

Doctor:

-You do not have anything, you'll be a lot better soon, and then you can go home.

Fikret:

-Ohh.Thanks..

-Allo ... Mother! I'm in the hospital.

Mother:

- What's wrong, son?

Fikret:

-I do not feel good at all, I thought I had a heart attack, but it was not.

-I do not know what it is, but the doctor said I can go home soon.

Mother:

-Okay, call me when you back home.

Fikret:

-Okay, I'll call you mom.

Fifty minutes later, the filled Diazem bottle was over and after Fikret extended a little longer,then he got up and dressed on.. after skipping a taxi he returned to home ,with clothes, he rested on his bed and fell into a deep sleep. As his eyes slowly opened in the morning, he woke up watching the smoky picture on the Wall. It took a long time to get out from bed. He reached into the cigarette pack at the head end and took a cigarette out of it and burned it.

Fikret:

-What happened to me yesterday? I thought I was going to die.

- I'm starting to get old! Fortunately I feel better today.

While Fikret was trying to figure out what he was living in, He was unaware of experiences he would have under the consciousness of which he would live with these Forbidden loves, the drugs he used, and thousands the anxiety episodes . When he starting out from the thoughts,burned his fourth cigarette.He was peskish and headache..

Fikret:

-I should go out and eat something and come to myself, I feel very tired myself.

-These streets, buildings, how beautiful was it before, our building was built in 1980. My grandfather had come here in the his youthful. I came to here the age of 37 as his grandchildren. .There were 20 flats in this apartment.I was knew all owners.Now I see that I have only to 4 flats owners knew from those years.Now there are no trace from my childhood friends who lived in these apartments. Everyone was scattered somewhere.

- How fast is the time passed? When i was a child i planted a seedlings here ,that saplings are branched,the leaves of tree were everything around me.My friends filled the leaves.But the time passed so quickly,All the leaves were poured out every autumn,then they built on this apartment.Whats that? The tree now fade away..I've just realized.I'm going to plant a new seedling right away tomorrow.Should come into leaf immediatly..And fill with new people..

Fikret:

-Bro two cheese pies and a big cup of tea! Please..

Baker:

-It is coming now..

Fikret:

- I do things so beautiful for people,always they are attacking me because they can not wait for these things to happen and they are very impatient.When I finalize these things myself and they become even more hostile to me when they see it.

- Maslow has made a very good classification,thanks him..

-For example: It would be nice to put together a panic attack patient, Borderline, Bipolar and Schizophrenia, and watching their speech and behaviors.

-We would produced a Community Disorder that all of them created. I think Social Psychology also needs medical support. What is a psychologist?I dont understand..

-Social Disorders, Community Diseases. This is racial and culturally distinguishable.. There is a savage society in the world. Everyone is crushing, destroying, destroying. Too brutish..The world culture is very dangerous like a monster. How people cause to forget each other to death!..

Fikret:

- My brother, what is my debt?

Baker:

- 8 lira

Fikret:

-Well ...

-Good luck Black Sea guy.

Baker:

- Thank you.

Fikret did not want to call anyone, he slowly started to walk to the governor's mansion street, when he came to the Teşvikiye Mosque, he took the cigarette packet out of his pocket and took out a branch cigarette and fired. He looked around and started smoking his cigarette. In the Nişantaşı's yellow greens,he began to walk, tilting his tired head in front of him, After entering one of the Cafe-Shops and taking the filter cup, he sat down on one of the corner tables and dived internet on his cell phone.

Fikret:

- Some moments and eloquent thoughts always dissipated..What a crazy World this..

- Perhaps it was dream of escape from every slap to your soul of dying consciousness.. Perhaps it was a condonation to speed up reaching this consciousness.. Thats all about it,all meetings,all look happy in the fake love rooms.

- Get close to people, get in their way and win their trust and break them down and smash them.

-Thank God! I have a hole to hide.

Fikret had been drinking too much coffee and sun has sunk..That deep darkness began to cover the city..As if all eyes was on him,everthing,everyone seemed to be following him.. He was strached to much,and too much ,He no longer had the courage to look into anyone's eyes.Everywhere, every moment, it starts to come fearful .

- Why is this guy looking at me?

- What are you following me?

- Or will you attack me?

- He wants to kill me?

- I'm going to get out of here right now and take a breath.

Fikret had forgotten his coat and ran towards the house with his running steps,it was coming all over town on him..even though his throat had dried up and he did not even come to his mind to drink water. He did not even remember how he came into the house... He reached into the couch, closed his eyes.He wanted to sleep but could not sleep..His eyes were slipping away..He lied for a few hours.

- I have to lock up everywhere.

CURE

- Who is this guy waiting in front of the door?
- Is he watching to my place?
- Somebody put somethings to my coffee ?
- My heart is jamming.
- I really think I will die!
- I have to go to the hospital right now ...
- I'm dying.
- My arms are not holding my feet.
- Alo, send an emergency taxi to Husrev Gerede and number 16.

Fikret was attacking again. This attack was heavier than the previous one. He was barely in front of the door of the apartment. The taxi driver was the same taxi driver.

Taxi Driver:

-Are you really all right?

Fikret:

-My brother, please bring me up to the hospital to American,

-I will die!

Taxi Driver:

- Stay calm.

They put to bed Fikret and tied Diazem to his arm.

Fikret:

-Doctor, tell me what do I have? I have heart attacks?

Doctor

- No, Mr. Fikret , we checked your heart is okay. You are having two days of worrying episodes. We are sending you to Psychiatry Department. You can go home when the serum end.. Tomorrow at 14.00, You have a date with Dr. Rahchan .

Fikret:

-Thank you so much .

Fikret, after end of serum got up and dressed and held home the way.

Fikret:

- This time I'm going on foot.

-So, Anxiety attacks ha?

-What's happening to you, Fikret?

- And this will come to you, beautiful soul?

- Anyway tomorrow I look at the doctor .. I will see how we will come from the superior of this anxiety. At least we are aware that disease..

- This awareness shows that I'm on my way ..

- What do these homos have to do with this street? Look at the stopping cars? Are you a man, man? This street has been a shit road .. run Fikret ...run!

-Ohh! There is nothing like own your house..I feel so good when I come here..I do not want to hear anything to talk about.I don't want anybody here..

Fikret was accustomed to lie down without changing his clothes. He was drowsy and suddenly filled the sun his room in the morning. He looked at the ceiling for a long time and threw the duvet in the place and awake..

-Dr. Rahchan! Does this solve it?

-Can you solve this Dr.?

- Then I can tell her what my whole life is like.

-You can solve..Yes you can..

-Fucken, bitch!

-How can it be that in this world of billions of people, people speak hundreds of different languages.How was that, brother?

- All the races came from different places to here?

-Look at it. Somebody's got a black , another slant eye, someone blond and blue-eyed.

- Look at the alphabet of the language they spoke to .. In Chinese ... Does this alphabet belong to the world?

-I do not believe .. Nothing is understood.

-God has expelled us from heaven. We do not belong here.

-All these tongues belong to the heaven... Were they there?

- I wanna break this mirror.

-Let's get out of here to yellow of the egg ...

Fikret had breakfast, he was very angry that he was getting sick, and he was ready to fight with somebody at any moment.

Fikret:

-Anyway, i wanna buy bitter chocolate .

- Do you have bitter chocolate ?

Grocer:

- Yes, there ...

Fikret:

- Why do you have it?

Grocer:

-Excuse me, I did not understand ?

Fikret:

-This one? ..

Grocer:

-Yes..

Fikret:

-How much ?

Grocer:

-3 lira ..

Fikret:

-Thanks..Good luck!

Fikret began to walk towards the hospital by eating chocolate.Then, he came to the front of the hospital. He saw the benches right next to the entrance. He saw the benches right next to the entrance. He looked at his watch,there were more forty minutes.

Fikret:

- I can smoke a cigarette over there.
- They say quit smoking and they produce billions of cigarettes every day.The person's head is all messed up..If it not good why you making big bazaar for this?
-I do not think about quitting.

-You must think about the children who died before, the children who are tortured, the people living in the world below the life limit. The weapons that you do not give up producing, the bombs are very useful health.ha?
-They are seeking nonsmoker ,for hard fucking!
-Anyway,its almost time..
-Dr.waits..
-She waits?

Fikret comes in from the hospital and comes to the counselor:
Fikret:
-Hello darling.
Girl:
-Hello, welcome
Fikret:
- I had a date.
Girl:
-Which department? Who did you have an appointment with?
Fikret:
-Psychiatry, with Dr.Rahchan ?
Girl:
-Ok, get out of here, get out to second floor, turn right, and you're in.
Fikret:
- Thank you..darling..
Girl:

CURE

-Bye

Fikret walked up the stairs, turned to the right, then came to the psychiatry department.

Fikret:

- I had an appointment with Dr.Rahchan.

Boy:

- What's the your name, Sir?

Fikret:

-Fikret, Fikret Demir.

Boy:

-Yes, sir, please wait right here, soon the lady will take you.

Fikret:

-Thank you..

Rahchan:

- Fikret ..

Fikret

- Yes ..

Rahchan:

-Come my baby ..

Fikret:

- My baby? What a touching voice it is. What a voice tone. I'm very impressed.

Rahchan:

- You can sit here ... Tell me what happened?

Fikret:

- How do I get started?

-Now I'm started to find myself in two nights in the hospitals,My heart starts to strike, i have hand and arm numbness, my throat is dry, I can not breathe and I think I will die.. It feels like everyone is looking at me as I walk on the road, I can not drive car..i think that always someone following me, I can not stop in my place. I always want to get away from somewhere. I can not work, my private life has come to an end. I know there is a problem. I have had this since years, but I never paid attention until 2 days ago.

- I am aware of what you are now, and I want to straighten it out and return to normal life.

- Actually, I can imagine why this is a little bit. I had lived in Russia for the first time. I had a lot of pressure on it and I was drinking vodka every night. It was hard to get out on the nights. Some nights I thought some people would come forward and attack us. I had a lot of similar things. A few years ago, they gave me something I have never seen in my life to drink in a very strange in the Christmas party, and I have swallowed it without asking. It seems that things started after that day.

- I think DMT is releasing this substance only when the human brain is born and when it is dead. According to the first time I was born, the second time I had secreted it through this substance caused me to have a like death process..

Rahchan:

-It could be..I saw..Now I will write you a few medicines, you will get them regularly every day. Our primary goal is to control the negative thoughts and doubts in the head. Come back one month later and let's talk and decide what to do.

- I wrote you Paxil, you will get it in the morning. I also wrote Seroquel, before you go to bed at night. This is my card, I have my cell phone there.You can always reach me at this number.If I do not give a reply, give me a message.

Fikret:

- Okay, thank you very much.

Rahchan:

- Come on, get well soon..

Fikret took a prescription and examined it for a while. After a long look at Rahchan, he left the room and held the path of the pharmacist. He entered one of the pharmacists nearest to the hospital and took his medicines. Then he entered a markete and took a water bottle and took the pills. He was deeply troubled by the thought of how he came to the cage he sat in.

Fikret:

- I'm gonna get rid of this disease in the shortest possible time, I'm going to pierce everything that's causing you.

- Let's see if these drugs work.

Tolga:

-Fikret!

Fikret:

-Ha! Tolga? What news, pal?

Tolga:

-Fine, what are you doing ? How many years?

Fikret:

-Fine, you ? Sit down?

Tolga:

-Let me sit down, I'm drinking coffee, and I ...

- Is it too much?

Fikret:

-Yeah, Tolga, it's been seven years since you kicked me out of the house for Sveta.

Tolga:

-What?

Fikret:

-Yeah..

Tolga:

- I did not kick you. You paid for what you still do or did you pay?

Fikret:

- Yo, I came to you, when I came, your fiancé had taken over you, you were in a state of bitter, sorry, you were very upset about this. And since I was very sorry, my friend, and said you that i will meet you with a girl

- And said you that :Just hang out with this girl for two or three months and then I said send her .. You did what you did, and I kicked me from the your house to seize girl for a year.

- Now you are charged me? Are you God Tolga?

-Ahh ... God punished me..

Tolga:

-Fikret ,you told me that :You can get marry to this girl before you left, and you told to me you did not do anything with this girl. Then You told me that you slept with this girl.

Fikret:

-Tolga it's your occupation, when you saw your to this girl and you forgot of your fiancée everything and about me. So you did not be clean neither to your fiancée nor to me. I told you these things about you so you do not have a lot of things with the girl. She slept with all my friends all the time in college. ..

Tolga:

-You Fikret know what you are doing now .. You asked me for money for this...You've infected me with the foolish girl.

Fikret:

-Well, was fine when you lay down with foolish girl for a year?

- I know exactly what I'm doing. Look at it. God is talking. What do you think of yourself, you are an angel?

Tolga:

-The real friend speaks always true Fikret!

Fikret:

-You are going to take off as a lawyer for these prostitutes, and punish me for the price?

Tolga:

- I'm not a lawyer.

Fikret:

-Why? Do you think you're an angel or something? If I had known, I would have wanted more money.

-Okay,we can close,You are not a friend of mine, you have such a deeply humorous flair in you that if you go out together with the war, you will be bullied in the back because of this banality.Now you can take your cofee and get off the desk.

Tolga:

-I m going Fikret

Fikret:

-Go, remember that you owe me an apology.

Tolga:

-You are Fikret!

Fikret:

-What am I? Come on, fuck off!

-Look at them..The world is turning around them..They are always in the most right places,always good, others always wrong and unfair.What a beautiful world!

-Go away!

Fikret took a cigarette from his pocket and fired his cigarette after he got out of the street. He put his headset in his ears and started listening to 'Boom Pam -

Tamid Levad.'He came home and extended his feet. Paxil was good. He was feeling relaxed and feeling more courageous. It was going to be a long time to come home and it would only be for food and necessity to get out of the house. He took medicines for days and started to spend his time listening to music on the couch. He was started to watch all the seasons of the foreign serials one by one. He was only communicating with the Rahchan on Whatsapp, actually with Rahchan who created it in his head. The real Rahchan was responding very little to his messages. Anyway, what Fikret wrote was not the kind to answer.

CURE

Fikret:

-Hello Rahchan..

-I was in Thailand. I have turned back a few days ago. I have overweight fatigue. I have a feeling of lack of willingness and motivation. I think it triggers seasonality. It is like depressive.

- How can I raise this ..? You said you can start to Efexor. I get Efexor for 10 months. In the last 6 months, 37.5 mg..

- Zero attack.

- My appetite is very clear.

- Just always i wanna sleep

-I could not come to you

- So this illness, in this seasonal transition could be to high but we have took this under control..Its just make me very fatigued..

- It's like this until the temperature difference between day and night is getting closer..

- I think there are so many people in the box like me !!!

Fikret:

- :)

- Coca Cola

- Did you read the book?

- Coke and canabis can be used for certain medicine.

- I talked to Mor and she said that you were not here.
- Exactly
- You're doing well
- Do not tamper..
-;)
- I will buy a car..

Fikret:
- Did you come ?
- I started with a Russian woman
-)
-I'll ask you something .. if I want to do a baby, do I have to stop taking these medicines?
- Does Efexor break the quality of sperm?
Rahchan:
- You do not have to quit.Women must quit.
Fikret:
- OK..

- Did I tell you that I made the master's degree in Russia and stayed there for 5 years?
- I am sending you a letter:
-Tesla said : About Over-sensitization of the his five senses and the troubles caused by this :
"The roaring sounds coming from far and away dragged me into fear.. And I could not distinguish what they were like. When sun rays periodically cut off, created such a great force on my brain and I was passing by myself. For pass under a bridge or something like this,i

had to push to all my volition,Because I was feel unbearable pressure in my skull.
- Nikola Tesla personally talks .. what will you think?
Rahchan:
 - Panic disorder

 Fikret:
- Wow ...
 - Very important information ...
- How is it? If i were psychiatrist and I can send it to brain at 7.63 Hz. And I could secrete serotonin as much as the effect of antidepressant with the magnetic wave. I think that the brain that has already been damaged also has a wave.
- It's being done right now ...
- Wow
- I thought right ..
- Its applying this quantum to psychiatry
 Is not it?

Fikret:
- Hi ... I am trying to bring my friend to you. He has some social phobic cases, but I can not convince them.How do I follow a method?
-This my friend when will communicate with women ,he lives hard panic episodes and he cannot establish a proper relationship.
-And he is aware of this
- I will bring him to you in a way ..

-This guy for 15 years could not be with women..He has everthing but its big problem for him..

-I did tear oneself away from Mor.. She was a woman who used spiritual feelings and tried to make people pay for themselves under friendship.

- Apart from that, it took 6 months to get rid of all the harmful ones with the same character.

- Those who manipulate the human being are actually just the ones who are near by us..

- When i crossed from Xanax to Paxil and Seroquel, she had not even warned me about this girl.. and she did the same thing in London. She gave me a name of her girlfriend, then she did not give her number ... She was shocked to when i met with this girl at Beymen Cafe..

Yesterday I got an e-mail from her : 1 year ago I mentioned her girlfriend about my painting,so think so she is annoyed to Şükran and then Şükran said her that i want from her to my painting..Mine says that i will send you to your painting..at that case she can brig it to you ok?

-I can take this from you..

- Take it away

- : Is it OK?

- My friend Levent will call you ..

- He will make an appointment and come to you..

- I gave him your phone number.

Rahchan:

- Ok,Fikret..

Fikret:
-Rahchan,Good morning..at Monday..
-When you are available?
-I will come to you..
Rahchan:
-Wait i am asking!
Fikret:
-Ok..
Rahchan:
-at 13.00

Fikret:
-Ok,i saw
-See you..
Rahchan:
-See you..

Fikret:
- I am here..
- : Nomad, rider of the ancient east
   Nomad, rider that men know the least
   Nomad, where you come from no one knows
   Nomad, where you go to no one tells
- I tell you an error that women make: when they realize that a man is showing interest ...its their retreating..It

becomes obvious that it is strategic and the event is losing its naturalness!

- Prozac input gave good reaction
- Efoxor was exhausted but he answered correctly.
- Are you able to read out the watermelon
- Arabic writing?
- Yes ,written Allah on the melon
- Jesus loves you
- Fantastic things are happening..

Fikret:
- Prozac: I woke up in the morning super .. I have not woken like this for long time..
-If Mor is naive ..then i m a brilliant..
- Prozac: drives out the consciousness of the past. Is this a sign that the area in which the unconscious is loaded is beginning to erase?
- Much of the past revives in my mind more in detail
Rahchan:
-This is not Empirical data..Fikret..
Fikret:
- I understood ... its like the flashbacks etc. when I drank
- Forgotten records are coming out.
- I got it.They are Repressed datas..
- Actually ... the data that unnecessary to be collected ... ike the cookies in the computer.. during the data connection ..hidden garbages...when it starts to take up

a lot of space .. it can make a ridiculous image as it wants .. it can be nightmare .. or it can be fantastic dreams .. We can argue ...
- I think root pain behind the eyes is the result of this.then headache and weakness..
- Prosac very good invention.
- Efexor is really a full system drug ..Fixed system ..
-Efexor is operating in the brain...
- All my Russian memories are bursting today :)
- Russia was completely erased before..

- : Хочу сказать что я очент хорошо имеею писать на русском ..:))
- : И могу говарить очень хорошо ..сколько девушек было у меня не могу считать..

- I have not forgotten
-Sorry Rahchan,I am harassing to you on Whatsapp for a few days ...I do not know if you believe it or not: I want to say that Prozac 's rapid entry and control of speed Is very effective with watermelon..
 - I've harassed 6 more people including you :)
- But: I'd like to congratulate you, and I'm to beat my panic disorders ...
- When I look at this picture last year, it seemed funny. But now there is very little minimum movement. You can use it with those experiences like using Lsd etc etc;)
- When I hear the bad word, I run away
- :)

CURE

- Efexor's fall effects are over today

- My dear Xanax is better than Prozac
- I will throw Prozac on the weekend. I will take Xanax in 2-3 days.
- Then continue without medication. Xanax will stand in the corner ..
- It was not come well?
- Apperantly..
- Yes, Efexor was good, but I will be out of antidepressants ...
- Sometimes I only can take Xanax ...
- Its revive you too much?
- How Prozac is: it fools you so much and makes you dizzy.
- Rahchan:
- Interesting..

Fikret:

- It is pleasant but does not arrange the thoughts locally
- Why is it interesting?
- I will not drink anything..what i have in my brain will go out.. I will check all..

- What I need: Efexor's awareness Xanax's blend of aphrodisiac effects on the ailment. Venlafaxine + alptosalum. Announced to biochemist friends. Panic disorder bipolar and anxiety They will find a breakthrough treatment in their treatments. Paxil, Prozac, Lustral, Rispardel etc .. all missing drugs ... There are those who do not want to stop the sales of pharmaceuticals I understand from here !!

- In this context I would recommend you to read this article

Fikret:

- Human Brain and Entogens - Tryptamine Derived Entogenes:

The living things are actually a reflection of the strange attractiveness of classical chaos theory. It contains living things that seem to be well-organized, and a chaos system that will encompass the entire universe. Therefore, as the beings discover their inner selves they discover the universe. Inner discovery is the convergence to the universe, that is, the universe. In this respect, it is not necessary to go too far to understand the secrets of the universe. In discovery of ourselves, the greatest challenge is to get rid of patterns and boundaries. Even if we get rid of all kinds of cultural pressures, we need some help to overcome biological barriers and communicate with the energy that surrounds us. This has been given to us by plants throughout human history. Those plants that we can define as consciousness are called psychic or entogenous plants. By creating change in consciousness, they experience experiences that are defined as spiritual and mystical. Since this is a discovery process, it is possible to get tired of many different things at first. But over time, this mystic and spiritual point of view leaves its place to the workings of the universe.

It is the basic effect of the development process of the human mind, psychic. Particularly consciousness formation and self-awareness, and therefore awareness, are an advanced process with the use of psychic materials. However, within the process of repression and manipulation based on the control that communities later enter into, the state of self-discovery and consciousness ascension is unfinished and even declined. The interesting thing is that people are encouraged to use alcohol, cigarettes, sugar, etc., instead of harmful psychic substances, to the dominant groups.

Human beings can not attain a complete state of high perception without herbal psychic materials that will enable one to reach its nature and nature. It is impossible for us to discover the world and the universe with only five senses we use on a daily basis, because that is not the purpose of the development of these senses. But with a real look we can understand our world, which requires freeing the brain. We are all part of a conscious mind, but we are not even aware of it. Very few of us are aware of this whole consciousness and trying to understand it, because taboos and prohibitions are preventing it. For example, these constraints have played a very important role in the development of human consciousness, on the basis of the explorers called shamans, and the communities that saw the world's real functioning. Shamans are also the ones who have reached the reality, that is to say, both sona and beginning. Thus instincts and the brain have been able to advance from a higher consciousness to a higher level of consciousness. The sharing of these experiences with society has made it possible for cultural and conscious structures to become more universal. Shamanism is not a religion as it is known. It is an experience that involves techniques that are based on the use of the world and the universe for exploration. It is the discovery of facts, there is no fixedness, it is based on keeping up with the changing world and discovering it. Psychological subjects here open the limits of perception. When these boundaries are opened, no one can close their eyes and mind to the press, to the control of society, to unnecessary destruction of living things, to the crushing of women, and to anything that does not conform to the true nature of man. The shaman acts here as an explorer, leading to the opening of human eyes. The basic message that nature gives us is dud, follow the dance of the universe, get rid of division and unite. Because the essence of everything is the same, and it is the whole itself. In order to capture the rhythm of the universe, the brain, that is, the mind needs absolute freedom, which in turn leads to a free and integrated knowledge of the facts.

The most important obstacle in the process of human liberation is the society and state structures that dictate what is right and wrong. In particular, the states manipulate and offer knowledge, religion and other means to people as support for their orientation and oppression. But this pressure does not last forever.

Humanity needs to be reborn. As a part of the cycle process of the basic functioning of the universe, mankind will return to the times when they can still live together and free, thousands of years before. This is an inevitable phenomenon. Even if people's brains are controlled, their molecules do not allow it, even if their molecules are controlled, they do not allow atoms, even if their atoms are controlled, the basic energy that connects us to each other is not allowed. . However, to hear this call of the universe, the boundaries of mind must be abolished with psychic experiences to comply with this rhythm. Otherwise we will be condemned to an eternal bondage and we reject ourselves. This brings with it unhappiness and pain. The part of mankind that is faced here is equipped with all kinds of economics and manupillation power, and they apply all kinds of plans for people not to wake up. We live in an era when societies are kept in touch with television, media and consumption. These are real drugs. Drugs direct people without giving them a chance to control. The psychic, or conscious, items hidden from human beings, on the contrary, are the linkers that help people discover themselves and the universe. People are like the car that takes them to the places they look for. This is what pressure groups do not want. Why is psychic stuff not legal? Because it poses a threat to society, if it is a threat to women's rights to obtain and how to express their opinions clearly is a threat. The dominant idea with this idea is unfortunately far from the truth. For thousands of years many cultures have found their way through the use of plants. We need these plants to guide us thousands of years in order to raise the level of consciousness, to live in a peaceful and free world.

Many plants have used it for many thousands of years during cleavage activities. However, some of them have had lasting effects on human intelligence and consciousness, and their places are separate. Especially the plants which contain the substances of the tryptamine origin come first. Plants containing the DMT (dimethyl-tryptamine) and silosybyne (psilocybin) substances derived from tryptamine have been used by many communities for a long time. These substances, which are used to reach conscious and changing experiences, are taken through plants. As a result of thousands of years of experience, people use plants that have proven credible. Silosaybin is found in many species of mushrooms and is used in rituals by people in Asia, America, Australia and many other parts of the world. DMT is found in many plants, but when used with MAOI (mono-amine-oxidase inhibitor), which is another herbicide, it has a very strong endogenous effect because it is rapidly destroyed in the body. DMT and MAOI are found in different plants and within these ancient cultures have managed to bring these two possibilities together in the forests of thousands of plants. In South America, a psychodynamic drink called Ayahuasca is prepared from plants containing DMT and MAOI. The structures of both DMT and silosaybin are very similar to the neurotransmitter of serotonin in the human brain. DMT is also a chemical normally secreted by the body. However, DMT is a dangerous "drug" in category 1 in international regulations. So our own brain is dangerous and forbidden. I leave the debate about why our eyes and the irrational material are forbidden, instead of drugging them.

Entogenous plants exhibit hallucinogenic activity. Hallucinations are the doors to reality that we basically escape. Hallucinations and dreams are situations in which the creature listens to itself and is far from external stimuli. It is the sense that the perception of the brain is clear, against the frequencies that the body carries by its own body. This means that the frequencies created at the quantum level, even at the lower level, can be perceived by the brain. The hallucinogenic state can be entered with many substances, but especially those derived from tryptamine are different. Because it is entered into a more intense and visual hallucinative state. The strong, light-filled universe enters the code world. There is a lot of information to be solved and followed. Many scientists are searching for the secrets of the universe far and in mixed ways. However, those who are experiencing many shamanistic and shamanistic experiences in the world, but who are called "magician or madman" in "modern societies", dominate the secrets of more universes than most scholars. Because they have seen that the koskoca universe is already in us and that communication with reality can be done through an inner journey. However, the important thing here is to be able to distinguish reality. Think about it, a very nice music is accompanied by a loud noise, you are listening, you are listening and you are trying to distinguish the music from inside. Therefore, it is up to us to discover the place where entogenous substances do not treat like drugs, they are the connection ways. These ways actually lead us to the heart of change. So we can see times that we have defined as past. We encounter a lot of information from the formation of the universe to the way it operates. It understands that the human brain is a part of a very wide level of consciousness, basically free from its borders.

It is difficult or even impossible for someone who is experiencing DMT experience to understand this experience. So, mostly these people live calmly in their own circumstances. Especially those who have reached the level of being a shaman can perceive the people very well. Because the levels of consciousness have been able to perceive the frequencies that people have been able to perceive.

- Do you think I can start study neurology after this time?

- Lycopene, PHOSPHORUS AND IRON.

- The point where hang out in my head: when the drugs are made abroad ... could the production in fact be made in Turkey, it would be much more reliable to find the right medicines .. When did we look at the history of the panic attack? Where it started as a localization .. how and how it spreads .. I do not doubt much about water and beverages .. I look at the years 70's panic is not even nobody pronounce .. period hippie periods ..

- And finally: I say societically, because humanity has undergone an evolution of biology, such abrupt sub-diseases are emerging. Will the generation that will emerge after 50 years from now will be biologically much more advanced?

-Now,when i have headache,i take Vermidon then my headache passes,when i have stomache ache ,i take drugs and my ache passes,but for my brain what i take..do not passes..Psychiatry should be the solutioner now..make something please..

- As of May 20th i left Efexor .. I left Prozac which I used between 16-26 May. I take only 0.12 mg Xanax per day and I feel super feeling my life.

-I started updating myself every day! I have been released for 3 years

- Healing healing ...

- Completely organic nature with love from mother earth

- :)

- I hate chemical industrial products..

- The side effect word is very noticeable.

- Make me your assistant, let all the patients turn their minds back to life :)

- I started watching TV, before never watch it ..

- I think we should bring a new clean antidepressant to Turkey?

- I can make it feasibility

Rahchan:

-Yes

Fikret:

- : OK

- I'm starting work on this..

-Which disturbances generally i should concentration?

Rahchan:

-Efexor-sized drug is needed without side effect.

Fikret:

- : OK ! Good choice

- Efoxor is very close to .

-Rahchan:

-You look on TMS business

Fikret:

- okay..

Rahchan:

- American will take for me.

Fikret:

- Ok What is TMS full opening .. Is there a specification?

Rahchan:

-We need to choose

-With navigation

-Brainsite navigation

-Transcranial magnetic stimulation.

Fikret:

- Oookkk

- Now it was super..

-All right, I will get the representation that I will hit the money !!!

Rahchan:

-Jewish brainsway, but the use of difficult instruments

-Magstim

-There is

-Magnatech

-Neurostar

Raschan:

- I know these

-But Germans also produce

Fikret:

- OK: I'll find out!

Rahchan:

-And nerve vagus stimulation

-Non invasive remote

Fikret:

- Done

- Goodbye to pharmacologists, it will groundbreaking ...

Rahchan:

-In 20 years yesss ...

Fikret:

-There is something that flees in mind: in fact, the ability of the brain to fix itself ... something that needs start up this from the outside. I think that the work that has been done is local area work ... a substance or signal, etc. the brain's self-repair and maintenance unit's power If you can turn the button on and off, you will scan your own, find the problem and fix it ... then it will continue on its normal path ...

- You need to see or do this in the following way. to hypnotize to person for too long. maybe 4 -5 more days !!

- I believe that this feature is in the back of the left brain in a region where the is cerebellum and medulla oblongata!

- So Cerebellum!

- Parkinson's disease can also be treated here. All the care of the brain can be operated from here.

-It is very interesting that there are hundreds of time slots in your brain. This abstract thing inside the brain is not tangible but it is not visible but it can be used ..

- Turkey is going to be macho ... what they will do with Cerebellum? :))

- So, for example, to stabilize the time zone in which the secretion of serotonin is passed through the brain ... like does the replay key always return the same song?

- : My dear, please write down what I wrote in the future some of the events in the brain will be solved ,i m already open your mind..

- Actually, one day I will have to draw and explain

- The way to tell just the brains is not exactly true, and used technology too!Can you imagine that the brain surgeon neurologists and psychiatrists who have been working for 100 years should realize that the things they are dealing with are empty trash cans !!!!

- They must see that alternative medicine which is humiliated and not taken seriously is useful.

- Here is my dear whispering the name of the fake medicine master of the money's lords - Medicine - ...

- Simply brain tumor surgery how much money in American ?! Money money money..

- Greetings..

- The reason of that the decaying structure is existence based on the foundations of the natural science and Darwinist dogmas ..

- If they are doing very serious business, all medical scientists come together and make everything for human beings free for humanity! Everyone in the world should get to free of the doctor's service.

-Rotten .. all of these rotten ..

-Nowadays, if you wanna get marriage, they expect everything from you without your heart.. For once the system is rotten , works for money and segregationist..

Hostile to humanity .. It can not be the man who manages humanity. .. Suddenly The blood vessel can torn apart ... no identity on the other side will be valid.. Although the zeros in the account are unlimited

- Happy Birthday to you jazz ... I will not catch up to cake!

- :)))

CURE

Fikret:

- Hey, I treated that borderline girl very seriously for 1 month..but the mother-man, father-marriage crap prevented her own children's health ..

- Especially for Borderline disorder the free associations attracted to my attention..

- And detected that they are so intelligence ..

: I want to tell the in brain where the free associations are managed to borderline disorders..

- This is something like a sound card. After the sounds and words enter the brain, it creates the image .. but this fake images ,dragging to patient to unrealistic fictions .. by living it..if you realize that you can manage to control it ..

- I do not think there is a drug for this disorder.. I recommend using lsd!

- Kortex + substania nigra = stiratum> talamus = process of the inner clock of the brain ..

- Talamus = borderline disorders

CURE

- Broca area

- The place where the brain's internal clock works, you know the working area of the dopamine that you mentioned..

- We have previously touch on to time zones :(

- I do not know if you will believe ..: I have a friend who will come to you: the guy I have been diagnosed with social phobia since March: he told me that :I had to go to a doctor in Ankara and he said ... .. and I told him : when you will go to doctor,will write you Paxil, yes his doctor wrote to Paxil !!!!! Call ask them ... I've been working for 2 months with this friend !!!!!!!!

- Yes yes yes ...

- So

- Mechanism :)

-Making the final decision! This is already your awareness ...

- It is normal to do this. When the problem is not solved, the other side of the brain too gets worse, it goes up to till bisexuality and homosexuality

- Normalized gayness and lesbianism ..Modernism !Fuck them all..Devils..

Rahchan:

- Woohoo

Fikret:

- Yeaa

- :))

- Haha .. look at the file! .. the blonde on the right i liked her .. she is single?I would love to eat a bagel in Machka Park with her?
- Our Mor, is look like a nigger on your side :)

-Now,maybe she can like me..she likes SİMİT?What do you think? If she doesnt like SİMİT,i can or for her PİLAV-TAVUK ! I can not immediately disassemble to my golden heart for her!
-This heart is both gold and priceless ..
Rahchan:
-You are very funny
-I think she is very sweet
-And single
Fikret:
- Let's meet
- They also sell milk corn.
- It is beautiful .. Mor says that this girl too rich for you..
- Introduce us ,we can see who is the rich?
-Love or Money?

- What exactly does set body temperature? Who is the manage of this in brain?
- I'm discovering
- So which area in brain responds to the heat signals of the blood ?
- Body heat and panic disorder related!
- There are things related to the blood..

- I think for panic disorders should be done in blood analysis about body temperature!

- An attack can occur due to a problem in the body that consumes fast water.

- Which is the question of which side of the problem would normally cause more water loss?

- Rapid water loss on the side disrupts the body heat setting .. this signal is going to brain..then brain being alarmed,and heartbeats are accelerating..

-tak..tak..tak..the body is getting very hot..the brain is reacting..should set the water in the blood..

- Should know the values of the blood ,when hungry and satiated ..

- Hypothalamus cells

- Pituitary gland

- !!!!!!

- So the vezopressin should be secreted right ..

- With love ..

- :)

- This guy now deserved a SİMİT in the park of Machka :)

-Near by should have something on the liquid too ... I will now find the right nutrient for this vezopressine setting.

-We must setting to not serotonin,we must settting to vesopresin..

- I think that the distant panic disorders related to the kidney .. and excretion ..

- And result: You were right of dopamine!

CURE

- BANANA the first in this case..

- But I made my dopamine in my brain too up ... setting this for me to normal took my 4 years.

- Drug + alchol + sex

- Fucked my brain ..

- Schizophrenia depend on dopamine..

- I love you my dear thank you

- End: I taught to my brain dopamine secretion after succeed..

- The pituitary gland should receive a continuous signal to adjust the water rate.When pituitary gland can not take this signals,occur anxiety,panic disorder and bipolar disorders etc.I thinks so it depends on person..

-The man who releases the dopamine and vasopressin can heal the borderline and schizophrenia.(this is my own work). I have two psychiatric books and one that I have worked on the internet. I should work on the vasopressin. Is there no antidepressant like this?

-This is a big mark an era!

- What do you think

-?

Rahchan:

- Vasopressin in men

-Increase Bonding

-In women

-Oxytocin..

Fikret:

- What can be balanced with dopamine vasopressin

-?

- This is very relevant to the water in your body ...

- They will secrete the right hormones so that they do not lose water

Rahchan:

-Water and dopamine

-Connectivity

-I do not know.

I will Look

Fikret:

- OK ..

- Let's sit down and do it

- : Banana

- Effective

- How about when the car overheats?

Rahchan:

- I will look ..

-I will return to you ..

-okay

- I think we should also write Efexor to Mor for a while ... to make sure that her age is 56 and that 20 year-old men will not want to enter into a serious relationship with her and to look carefully at the mirror.

- I do not think pedophilia should not be out of awareness.

- pedophilia!

- She seriously needs to have a macho who will envy her very much and show her this ... I think this jealousy to Mor will satisfy ...

- If you are careful, I do not call sexuality.Jealousy!

- With Love..

- In older women, jealousy, extreme jealousy can reach a paranoid point ... that's why they cries for love ... It seems like a obsession ... I've tried to before with a woman 10-year-old then me .. That time I was reading Frued,Women can feel like nothing at all without jealousy. So they can make deviant relations .. they can have vengeance weapons against their partners ..

-Questions of there is someone else and like that paranoid minds can leading them to other relations..and they can cheat their partners...It is impossible for a man to sleep with a woman for 10-20 years without stopping . it seems like make too much kids so sensible..Temporary orgasms and obsessive distorted sexual relationships.The older woman's brains that to see her young.Serious trauma!

- Sexual hunger!

- So the orgasm of a woman over 40 is jealous.

- With the same woman man's desire is diminishing..Its same for women too..

- Let them continue their efforts to find rich husbands. They should not end up spending. If they are in their early years, which type of brain they have i can noot understand..

CURE

- In the streets there are lot of Superman and Batman..The hero saviors javelin in the streets :))
- Beauty that can not accept death and despair .. Beauty is unfortunately not infinite ..

Rahchan:

- in Macka park
- And the banana
- I think I stayed there...

Fikret:

- Let's stop there, what is that friend's name?
- The sweet girl on the right in the photo blonde one ..
- Banana leads us in the dopamine system
- I would like to have a woman like you in my life.
- Name is important

Rahchan:

- Talya

Fikret:

- Russian?
- Russian name

Rahchan:

- Azeri.

Fikret:

- I went to Baku 3 times
- Their girls are strong
- What she doing .. I know Azerbaijanese
- Rahchan:
- They have vodka and wine factories

Fikrek:

- Then the religion phenomenon is different
- No, this girl not for me
-!
Raschan: Mor will introduce you ..
Fikret:
- No no
-No,Mor ok?
- Thank you
- I kissed..
-I dont like wine and vodka..
- I want a lady with a blonde, a neurologist from hospitals or like a neurosurgeon ..I can eat with her SİMİT in the Machka Park..Or i can drink with her Turkish Coffee around Karaköy .. a surgeon woman is my first choice .
- I need some serious brain-blown female brain to me .. I do not need the pieces of paper between the two legs and the wallet .. I have a wonderful allergie especially for the female who is drinking raki .
- The baby that I will bring to the world must shake the world from the place ..
- Today's our subject is potassium
- You need to laugh
- My dear you must laugh
- Meanwhile I ordered a cadaver
- Brain cadaver
- Not human
- :)

Rahchan:

- Let's laugh

- : Best of

- There is no such thing as making fun of yourself..

- If I had a chance, I would like to have a look at the cerebellum ..

- Why: because the brain will repair itself from here.

- Is it necessary to clear the blood in your body every year, or is there any other way of renewing the blood?

-?

- I entered the brain surgery subject very hardcore ..

-Normovolemic Hyponatremia !!

- Banana.. banana.. my dear ..it is a potassium phenomenon !!!

- Fearful my dear fearful have it made Cocktails in all the hormones secreted in the brain..

Rahchan:

-Wow

-You are writing Strict Things

-Bravo

Fikret:

- Do you want to see the whole book?

- 200 odd pages

- I will send you a nice song

- :)

- Cem Adrian interpretation

- Very cool beats in depth

- I can mix it.

- I will print the book, then I will make a hiphop album ..
- Style psybient hiphop..anatolian folk + electronic..solutions will wander from :)
- Eyes shoot with glances around ...
- This body will defend it until when
- I said I wake up the monster inside
- He started to look too hard..
- If necessary, vomiting every time will not be difficult
- :))
- Now I pull the video clip.
- I say the monster is looking around
- Condemn what: the poison of what people do not say and can not say
- The eyes will glance around like a bullet.
- Very cool beats in depth
- I can mix it.
- I say the monster is looking around

- The sympathetic pathway is derived from the hypothalamus...Tear source..Brainstem..The process until the tears stronger than blessed serotonin..
- First of all, we must fix to community health, then individuals...
- Very interesting, the tear goes out from the nearest point to the brain ..We can create placebo in the brain ,then brain automatically can feel self tearful..like that chemical formula can be effective..
- Love melancholia trip

- What they say : touched to my spirit
- This chemistry will touch to our spirit..
- Something to remember very well to people that they are human..
- These substances are present in MDMA components
- But must be made into tablets more tightly..
- Lets dance
- www.youtube.com/watch?v=QCzTnnLmm3w

- Plz watch very quality this:
- Hypnotic beats
- At last: www.youtube.com/?v=EtzDkS63ptA

- Frankincense!
- Did you hear this item
-This is a wonderful essential oil and I can cure some diseases by massaging this substance
- Its can improve quikly to Brain tremor and post-operative scars..
- It brought the seeds of the tree from Texas and did not accept soil that I planted in Mardin and the climate
- Desert climate is needed ..
- Plz check it..
- I was going to ask something about Biomechanic.
- https://www.youtube.com/watch?v=9bJB-adutY4
-I have 35 Boeing and Airbus aircrafts,and we have 8 jet and 5 helicopters.I am looking for a serious business man who can sell them.

- I need a wife like the woman at the head of the IMF
- I have one problem: everyone works very slowly I am fast ... I solve fast, others slow ... This slowness is preventing me from doing all..

- Now in the Pierre Loti ice cream could not be bad :)
Rahchan:
-Fikret
-I tought you are disappear

Fikret:
- :) i worked too hard..
- But the reward will be huge
- I'm hanging out without drugs
- Fuck off all crooks..

Fikret:
- I'm telling someone something ... that person is trying to direct me in the other direction to make what I want to say.
- There are People who can not learn to listen
- I worked a little bit for blindness treatment..
- But this times i am so busy
- I can not give up Russian girls either
- The situation is good ..
- I clean to my blood with the banana + yogurt and nettle tea..

- And I make swearing every day for all the fake and evil people! ;)
- Happy holidays
- The most just woman in Nishantashi you are..
- God always protects you ...

"I never thought of taking revenge on my life, life is more creative than me."
Simone

Rahchan:
- Simone is the woman of special elections
-She has Revolutionary spirit, has tried to defeat.
Fikret:
-Yes she is ..
- I heard just from you that she Revolutionary ... but it's obvious that she wanted to get serious revenge
Rahchan:
-Relation with Sartre is revolution
- :)
Fikret:
- Lilith and Eve..
- Actually there are two kinds of women, one is Lilith and the other is Eve ..
- I think Lilith is mostly in France
- Women fighting with men
Rahchan:

-The woman's struggle with not being a woman

- This is a much better perspective

- I prefer Eve as a man

- Eve

"I am most forgiving myself for dreaming with people who will not be."

Camus

Rahchan:

- Camus!

-Right.

-Mea culpa'

Fikret:

- The only thing that really matters is finding your love and liking in the same way

- The rest of: the decor and streaming film strip

- Then she can understand that she is a woman ...

- Who knows how to love what is not loved! The number of those who are aware of this is low

- Master and Margarita ..!

- I recommend reading a great book

- Russian metaphysics fantastic

Rahchan:

- Thank you ...

Fikret:

- : You're welcome.

- Being a woman is really hard for a woman to accept it?

- If so, the situation is terrible!

- Do you know why? Because that time making a bonus for prostitutes! Very important subject
- When the woman is thinking about herself, the whore already starts to fuck the guys !!!!
- Look at , its my psychoanalys.

Rahchan:

-Certainly, such women should discover the power of being a woman
-Then everything can be change
-But in this day's woman are
- wants to be a man.

Fikret:
- You wrote wonderful words...
- Once women should notice How the birth is a crazy regeneration..
- You do not have to make too much effort to explore
- Do you have a child?
- So today's women are so useless
- Today's woman is Lilith
-;)
-The first you should open your heart then will open your brain..you should open your brain then will open your eyes..You should open your eyes then you can look to mirrors..

Rahchan:

-I have 2 kids

-There is..

-But it could have 10

- I would love to..

- It could have been great

Fikret:

- I know a woman gave birth to 13.

- At the moment she 108 years old.

-I think so who has 10 kids can not find a time for think that :who am i? what am i ?

-As a mother with ten brains around her..

- I think that the dictating system of modernism of gay, lesbianism and their analogues, both humiliating the human race and downloading large bumps into the reproduction of the human race. - I look at the families in America, most of them are 5-6 children .. very interesting ..?

- In the meantime, I am in Istanbul

- I would like to have a cup of coffee if available

- We are planning to set up an office

- : Soon...

- A wealthy woman who knows how to use money, she wisely can spend this..but a woman who get money owing to her marriage,will be such a pleasure to spend money..She can spend her money in a big splurge.

- do you any experience of epilepsy?

- Is epilepsy treatment healer in Turkey?

- I do not think there is a positive result

Rahchan:

-There is resistance epilepsy
-depend on epilepsy
- But again neuroemodulation results in good results.
-FDA approval soon
Fikret:
- Ok we can moot this topic
- There is a patient
- I will direct to you
- I will take care of it for a while ..

- I was able to talk to this epileptic patient for 2 hours..It was an interesting thing that attracted attention.He said that it does not fgood for him hot weather and said the cool air is good ... and i remembered of water in blood and body temperature settings,so : To Vazopresine.
- The body can not adjust the body temperature because of epilepsy
- Pituitary gland!
- Now, what is the difference between the magnetic electrical currents that occur when the hormones in the pituitary gland work in normal motion, and the magnetic electrical frequencies that spread when there are epilepsy or other disorders?
- These signals need to be equal to their normal state.
- So compare the normal values of the pituitary gland hormone release with the post-disease frequency values and convert them back to normal values.

- There must be a machine that can do this ..
- I came across today. The Turkish girl is 21 years old. She lives in the same room with a man who has the 12 year old son and the 7 year old girl from Germany. What the hell is this Rahchan ... They met with this Turkish girl on the internet ..
- Of course the man is German
- Completely sex head .. this 20 's girl I guess she can not keep a piss when she comes to her 50 's..

Rahchan:
-Do not tell me such things
-I'm sorry..
Fikret:
- Yea
- Life is very dangerous
- Brain shocks go down..
- Big disorder this works .. watch true detective
- Real
- The system created a monster
- Sad, I do not write these things again
- But I saw many things
- Today I developed something like the principle of compatibility.

Fikret:
- An attack came and went with love ...
- I can control

CURE

- Efoxor is exhausted and cleaned in my blood
- 60 days
- Full
- I can read books for a long time now ..

- Get well soon

- Hey Rahchan, how are you?
- I hope everything is okay

-Raschan:
-Yess..
-Are you okay too?
Fikret:
- Good ..Thanks God..
- I am in istanbul
- I settled in the side of the Harbiye
- Jobs.. I work too hard ..
- :)
- Social disorders now very hardcore
- Due to recent events, from extreme stress came up with 2 short episodes
- Is this meaning using Efexor again?
- There was a conflict in front of my house at night..
- I discovered paracetamol
- It works well for extreme tension and headaches
Rahchan:
- Take half of Dideral 40 mg

- Every day.

Fikret:

- Antidepressant?

Rahchan:

- Not

- Superbly, taken in extreme excitement and stress situations ..

Fikret:

- Ok i'll check thanks for advise ..

- Let's have a coffee one day

- I am in Nishantashi every day

Rahchan:

-I am not in of Thursdays and Monday.

Fikret:

- Ok when the times are right

- My teacher I can see you this Friday ... I will tell you some for your future .. look what you will think!

- Dideral is very good and calmed down. Thank you ..

- He is doing bad forgetfulness ..but it is also makes thirsty ..

- I have seen a big ego balloon: what do you think about of woman who opening up her legs to the end and walking like that on the Abdi Ipekci with her 15 cm heel?And that all the men who look at her and women are what got from that?

Rahchan:

-Failed coup!

Fikret:

- Very good comment
- Too funny
- I am at Cafe Nero if available come here..

Rahchan:

- I'm in the Bodrum ..

Fikret:

- Okay
- Next time
- Bodrum now awesome
- Do not return:) (
- Rahchan: I am Göcek

Fikret:

- Very good .. I am Akyarlar
  - I see in your fortune A university looks good
- : What is that?

Rahchan:

-My fortune

Fikret:

- Yes
- There is a boy
- and a key..
-From far away like that..

Rahchan:

-Oha
-Super
-Bless you..

Fikret:

- I do not look too much I looked at someone last year what I said she saw..
- Only for My close friend in a year once or twice ..

"The child tries to climb the shed; A benevolent man keeps it from the ground, sit on a branch. Regrettably, the child has been disappointed, never happy. Because he just did not want to be on top of the tree, he wanted to climb it. As you can see, there are such purposes, such good things thatIt can not take place when we intercept; Someone else can not get them if we help.. So, if there is something someone else expects from us, let just do it; Otherwise, we will not be doing anything at all."

Simone

Fikret:
- I rolled half-Xanax to wake up the sleeping design beast in my brain ..
- I start the day with 3500 m running .. I sweat my head .. :) I recommend it .. I can run by running sometimes as I play basketball days .... xanax trip of the cleanest :))

- Xanax ganja trips already..
- In principle I will find the right gang and drink will take it every 3 to 4 days
- I am removing the state of emergency inside of me :))
- Look at my dear :

"Boy:
-How are you my love?
Girl:
　' You're a bastard.You do not know how to walk with a girl.You made me disgrace to my friends.You do not know me how to walk beside my friends. When I do garbage trash, you cleaned it them .. Fuck you .. fuck off from my life .. you already make three pennies ..then you are coming to me and saying love you . I am seeing you cleaning windows every day in front of the school..I am not used to it like that..I miss the Selcuk..I was too glad to go to some nice places with him..We drinkonly tea with you..Bye..
Boy:
'I understood when my parents and my mother died. I have looked at my brothers and sisters. I took all for them, I gave all to them. Anyway, there is no need to stretch it. We are not a Selcuk, but we had a heart."

Fikret:
- It's always been a matter of extreme interest.
- The irrelevance can kill them ..
- So I only choise the Russian

- Gangesterism starts like this, says Fikret ..

- When talking, the words come out of my mouth and go to the brain from the other's ears, and then it is recovered ... As soon as the words pass in front of himself, they will show themselves. For this reason the person will be lost in importance for me.

- I said to a European : How u do ? he said that :you do not know english :))

- Haha..I said that I'm Turkish :))).

After months, Fikret meets with Rahchan:

Rahchan:
-Come on,sit down Fikret ..
Fikret:
- I have a black friend, can I bring him ?

- After you when we are walking with my black friend, I saw Mor and Elif in Beymen Cafe and Mor called us to their place .. .. Mor gave to us the wall..Said us that we we will come to Cafe Nero..Come there..I knew that she will send Elif then will come to us after 50 hours..Cos of noone loves her..She is evil..

- My dear she has not a heart like yours

- I did it intentionally,she is not change..

-Look to this photo..
- From Russia..We studied together with her.

- Sweety yea?

Rahchan:

-Yea

Fikret:

- Yes good

- I will go to the temple of Zeus tomorrow

- I will Climbing

- I will rear there the Turkish flag ..

- If Simone was there ,said that fuck society ... and she looking at the sea in the Sirkeci and smoked her cigaret .. The women should be revolutionary and populist and laborer.

- Today I have a sarcastic fondness .. but I can not hurt anyone ... is accumulating in side of me and accumulating ... Let's explode..

Rahchan:

-Une situation Dangereuse

Fikret:

- :)

- Yea..Cos of shoul write on papers

- L'avenir est un long passe

Rahchan:

-Already gone

- Yes, I can manage to stay positive

 Rahchan:

-Do not be Pessimist!

Fikret:

- Sarcasm is different

CURE

- There are someone those who deserve it.

Rahchan:

-Yes, of course.

-in spades

Fikret:

- Sometimes I just get in and out.
- I dont forgive
- I use it to raise awareness to the other side , so maybe they can come oneself and fix it ...

Fikret:

- Heyo ... greetings
- What kind of word is kokosh :)

-:))

Rahchan:

-A beautiful Word

Fikret:

- Good find
- Very good brand for quilt pillow bed linen set
- It can be good bar name in Nisantashi
- Midpoint goes and comes Kokosh

Fikret:

- I have good connections with the drug.
- Does it work if we bring in some medicine?
- They are doing very serious studies Biochemistry
- Especially is not psychiatry.

- I have affiliation problem

CURE

- There is
- Never want to be a permanent member in anywhere
- I noticed that
- No place belongs to the institution person etc.

- I have always escaped from pertain
- Can you say a single word about reading the mind is one of the best :)

Rahchan:

- Bullshit

Fikret:

- Not true
- Let's open a Russian hospital next to American Hospital..

- To brain enters data from outside. You can not see that..can not touch..
- What if we do see it?
- The rate of cancer in Russia is very low and in China
- Why Western countries are always fighting cancer
- They are making the disease..
- Then they make money on drug treatment etc.
- Look at the sector?

Rahchan:

- You're right
- A crazy mindset crazy really.

Fikret:

- I do not remember where I forgot my heart .. I absolutely lost it myself ..
- I started to reduce to my loads
- I had a lot of people on my back with their good loads
- I'm going to continue to my career again soon
- Fully institutional.

Fikret:
- Greetings from Russia..
- I saw you in my dreams ... my dear..
Rahchan:
-Yaa......
Fikret:
- Yeah
- I saw the Devil ..
 Rahchan:
-It was me?
-Oh my God..
Fikret:
- Finished to my book
- I will translate to Russian ..
- will Publish here

CURE

- Satan Mor works with devil not you !:))

- Do not tell her about me I completely removed her from the list..

- : Ok? I trust you.

- I got lot of time Frustration from her .. for a long time i wont be in Turkey .. greedy monsters and dinosaurs!

- A lot of greedy herd..

- I improved in 5 months this friend who has social phobia disorders in 5 months.

- I want to be alive like this .. Need to increase to my urge... I will take an appetite from life but I will not break libido ... because I do not use anything for a long time .. the energy is low ..

- A medication that will energize your system without disturbing the libido ...

- Or is it amino acid protein powder?

- :)

Rahchan:

-Wellbrutin

- 150 mg

- Increase Libido

Fikret:

- : OK

- Super

Rahchan:

-Exactly

CURE

- This is not an antidep?

Rahchan:

-Yes antidep..

Fikret:

- How long I should use this?

-?

Rahchan:

-Take a look.

Fikret:

- OK, when you quit not makes bad trip?

- I had not take Paxil for 4 or 5 days in Scotland;then was too bad..

- : Thank you

- Do you have a request from Russia?

Rahchan:

-No thank you

-Ah

-Ethnic patterned scarf..

Fikret:

- Ok..kept..i will bring when i will come to Turkey

- There are things like that

Rahchan:

-Russian girls wear..

- They are..

Fikret:

- :)

- Open this Belarusian flag, and look to patterns ,good?

- Manic depressive: depression emerges from the hatch

CURE

- This is the extreme melancholy on me for a week, i said: what is that?
- Wellbutrin 150 xl
- Really xl
- made high..
  - Let's see what happens in 1 week
- A comfortable medicine
- Recommended for a long time after Efoxor

Rahchan:
-Its not selling in Turkey..Now. Bring a few boxes if you need this medicine
-Please bring me one, please.
Fikret:
- OK
- After panic attack treatment with Efexor, may cause major depression and treat it with wellbutrin
Rahchan:
- Is it so ... ???
Fikret:
- She told me that
- The my ex-girl is and she is a psychiatrist

Rahchan:
-There is no such thing
-If I say
-Forgive my arrogance

Fikret:

- Ok no problem .. there are many fractional things on these issues.

Rahchan:

-Ok

Fikret:

- Partizan

- There is a very rich and bossed man who thinks himself a communist in our homeland

- Anarcho communism is exactly for me

- And there are lot of politicized artist

- They shoul to see real Kommunalka life?

- Welbutrin drives the kidneys ...

- :)

- I think one of the best antidepressants is Xanax..

- My body does not accept any antidepressant anymore

- A single Xanax occasionally .

- Life sometimes takes some inspiration from our depths and does not give it back for a long time

Rahchan:

- I think so you are During the incubation period.

Fikret:

- I am in a strange period yes.

- Very strange

- I say that Fikret coming out of it will get what he really wants

- It took too long, it is keeps going ..

CURE

- Did you read Dostoyevski's The Idiot?
- I know I have severe depression
- About 1 month more i got flu than I passed
- And I started sticking to the bed
- I can say how the extraction did not make it wonder
- Very interesting I've always been alive for years as energy ..
- Because I did not feel well when I came home
- I had a brief episode. After a stressful family debate ..
- I am very tired and tired and in a bad trip ..
- Override now..
- I will win
- I made a down up .. !!
- I want to have an electroencephalography and see if there is something that does not affect my eyes .. I want also see the psychological state of my soul ... and i got hypermetropia and astigmatism ... can we measure the visual acuity with electroencephalography?

Rahchan:

-We can not Fikret!

Fikret:

- OK
- I will take MRI ..please check it for me..
- I will send you to my brain mri result
- I return to Russia tomorrow
- With Love
- Unfortunately, I was born with a mental illness.
- Kiss

CURE

- Something to ask I was forgotten
- You are listening to everyone's problems, listening ... lots of info
- How are you?
- Do not you need to refresh yourself like this?
- Who will listen to you?
- : I will listen
- Maybe it would be beneficial for you
- There is little experience
- I think that you need to recharge
- Is that wrong?
- I thought you should break some chains in you

Rahchan:

-Yes i have my dear ...

-I find peace wit nature and my dreams.

Fikret:

- I understand ... If you have a time in the summer,you should go to Minsk ,40% of the country ..forest....perfect
- Oh ..if it were not dreams
- Rent a bicycle and ride between the trees.
- I will come one day to you .. I brought you 1 box of wellbutrin .. we will make you a head massage .. we will take your mind .. take care of yourself ..

- What do you think ..?I wanna back to Efexor!
- I have Low level attacks rare.. rare ..
- Its was good for me 37.5!

- Neither Paxil nor Prozac nor Welbutrin..Xanax has done good ..but Effexor has done very well me

Rahchan:

-Take to Efexor

- The same was very good because
- I will see you next time

Rahchan:

-Take and make it up 75 after 10 days..

Fikret:

- You say?
- okay
- But I did it ... then 75 came a little hardcore.
- I will do what you say I will fix it to 75 ..
- : OK

Rahchan:

-Try it

Fikret:

- i Remember that I made that 150 ,could not take, 75 was fast,after 4 mounths i quit from 75..and took 37.5..ok 75!
- Agreed

Fikret:

- Euro islamic paradox in our land
- Hagia Sofia: islamic orthodox.
- This boy Levent will come to you
- He said ..
- Now i feel very nice my self..Thanks Efexor!...Ooohh!

- The man is eating, I sit in front of him and I started to eat and conversation ... I raise the head and look at him ... He looked at me and said :why do you look at me like humiliating me ...
- A view how much be insulting? .. I saw he some schizoid points ..what do you say?
- Is this against me?
- :)
- Always Simone in my mind .. life is much more creative ..

CURE

- If we decide to stop the intervention as the peoples of the whole world ... after a maximum of 100 years everything is over .. then? A big gap and silence.
- Is it too destructive
- :)
- How would you doa painting of that? I would like to see!

Fikret:
- How r u
- :)
- Fxor is very good
- Slowly goes out depressed
- The head is very good, this pill is only sweating the first 4 -5 days of Mouthpiece and sleep disorder.
- Thirst
- In the prospectus mentions water retention
- As I said before, dopamin-water relationship
- Sec dopomine is not healty..cos of i do not use it
- But it is pouring hair.
- When people can not accept you as you are, you become someone else.

-And they always while talking to you you feel your self not like your self ... as long as this situation goes on, someone else really makes you other ...
- But you never want to be someone else!
- This is the only way to see how they want to see you..
- It was even tiring to play a role here
- Expectations and expectations
- The person or persons who make you someone else ,they can blame you as a other, that is, someone else, you do not want to be accused of being someone else
-;)
- Get out now as a child!

Fikret:
- Hey
- I knock the door, I thought you are :)
- Today is my birthday
Rahchan:
-Happy birthday ...

Had actually knocked on the door, almost never knocked on the door for more than two years, he had gone out of his way to get his food and needs at , and his conversation with people did not even last a minute.

Fikret:
-Who is it? it can not be Rahchan anyway...No...I dont think..

-Oh, Rahchan! How did you find me?
Rahchan:
-I got your address from Mor.
Fikret:
-Come inside ...
Rahchan:
- I was very curious, Fikret, I have read all of your messages for a long time, but for weeks it has not sounded, your phone is turned off. Luckily you are looking for your family. I am very worried.
Fikret:
- I got it. You're welcome, Rahchan.I m very glad..

Rahchan:
- Actually Fikret, I'm in love with you, now I want to live with you .. What do you think to live with someone like me?
Fikret:
-Why not, you are always the woman of my ideals ..
Rahchan:
-So, let's go, let's go somewhere out together and talk for a long time.
Fikret:
-No Rahchan, I feel so good at home, I want to continue painting ..look at them..
Rahchan:
- Come on, then I'll make you a coffee.
Fikret:

-okay...

Rahchan:

- By the way the house is very nice and big, but there are so few things, even the bed is on the ground ..

Fikret:

- I like purism.if you do not mind..

Rahchan:

- No, no, no.take your coffee..

Fikret:

-Thank you ..

Rahchan:

-Bon Appetit..

Fikret:

- Now, Rahchan... When did you decide to come to me and find me? Tell me what you feel .. This flower is for you ..

Rahchan:

-Thank you .. I felt very lonely in the past year, and you were writing very impressive things to me. At that time, these letters had been very good to me and I was deeply affected and a Fikret started to take part in my head. It grew bigger and bigger. .

Fikret:

-I understand ...

Rahchan:

-It was very impressive things, you shared the pain that you live.

Fikret:
-Yeah, there was a storm in my depths at that time.
Rahchan:
-Thank you for accepting me..
Fikret:
-Thank you so much for coming out here and telling me honest and most sincere clearly all that what you felt .
Rahchan:
-I believe I will be happy with you, Fikret.
-I want to hug you and kiss you.
Fikret:
-You smell so good ..

Rahchan:
-You too ..
-I want to stay here tonight, with you.
Fikret:
- if you feel good.Yes you can..
Rahchan:
- I feel so good with you ...
Fikret:
- I want to read a little something.
-You can go out and get your goods, Honey.
Rahchan:
-It's a good idea ... I'll be back soon.

Fikret sat in the seat in front of the window and continued to read the book . It was long time and almost finished his book.The door knocked again.

Fikret:
- Why are you so late? It is midnight, Rahchan.
Rahchan:
-Yeah, Fikret, I could barely recover, I had a lot of work to do.
Fikret:
- OK, come on in.
- It would not bother you to sleep with me in this bed, would it? Because there is no other bed in the house.
Rahchan:
-No..No Fikret ..I m happy with you..
-Come on, let's sleep, I'm so tired,
FikretÇ
- It's okay.

Fikret did not change his clothes and couched to bed ..and Rahchan to his bosom..
They hugged each other and quickly fall into dreams. Rahchan was watching the Fikret when they were waking up.

Rahchan:
-Fikret!
Fikret:

CURE

-Yes honey?

Rahchan:

-I saw you in my dream last night ?

- We were getting married. One night was strange. There was nobody around us. We were going to , a wooded place by the sea, the weather was so beautiful, the wind was blowing our faces in the shape of an internal heater. .

- Are you marrying me? You say ..

-I said yes.

-We were very happy.

- Do we that something like that? Do you want to? Let's have a marriage that noone does not know.

- Let's do it.

Indeed Fikret and Rahchan had found the place they were looking for exactly in the same day. Did Fikret see dream, or did he not see it, did Rahchan come or did she not come?

Fikret:

-Rahchan you are so beautiful, you marry me?

Rahchan:

-Yeah Fikret marrying .. Do you marry me Fikret?

Fikret:

-Yeah, Rahchan..

Rahchan:

-I love you. Thank you for accepting me.

Fikret:

-I love you too ..

Fikret was married to Rahchan, but never realized that he was not a real Rahchan. When he had gone out for a night, yes he really went out, he went to wooded places on the edge of the sea.But he did not go with Rahchan. The woman he married that night was a goblin..

He had spent his life with her for years . He spent fortty years of his life like this and he gave his last breath at the age of seventy-seven at the front of window where he read book. When started to smell his body, neighbours entered the house and encountered a lifeless body. There was only a sense of meaning, filled with thousands of meaningless paintings and signs drawn on the walls of the rooms.

Neighbors:
- What a strange man he was with everything, my neighbors?
Neighbors:
- Yeah, yes, he never talked, he did not get out of his house, he talked to himself for years. Look what he drew.
- His death is so strange, is it my neighbor?
- I never saw him go out in the daytime. I remember coming into the apartment late at night, but ...
- What did he do?
- He told me he was a painter.

- Looks like everywhere is full of paint and portrait.

- Was he a famous person?

- I really do not know. He never liked to talk.

- What do you think these tables will be?

- He has noone..

- Always he was alone.

- What's the next article? You can read ? Look..

- What does it say, under the eye in the picture resembling the sketchy female body on this wall?

- Maje? Majo ... Majes? MAJOR...

- Yes, yes, it says MAJOR.

- What does it mean, huh?

- Anyway, the cops are here.Lets go..

CURE

COMMISSAR

Ekrem:
- Halil!
Halil:
- Sir, my lieutenant.
Ekrem:
- Come on in here and take photos of all the letters and pictures on this wall ...
Halil:
- You ordered me, Captain?

Ekrem:
- Investigate the situation thoroughly, no details are out of sight.

Halil:
-OK..

Ekrem:
- What is this picture? I have never encountered such things in my life.
- Where's the body, boys?
- On the couch in front of the hall glass on the front.
- What business is he doing?

Halil:
- Captain, does not anyone know what you're doing?
- But the painter says his neighbors never leave the house.

Ekrem:
- I can see from the tables ... drowned quietly in death sleep.
- What is it on the wall? I could not read it:

'I took the key to my hands..
The door of that love
Answer silently to my voice
Will open my door to your heart ...'

Ekrem:
- It writes ... What is it?

Rahchan:
- Hey, do you hear me?
Ekrem:
- What? Who are you ? Where are you?
Rahchan:
- Its Rahchan..
Ekrem:
- Oh my God, what is happening ... I hear unseen sounds ...
-Calm down...
- Haliiil ... Immediate ... come here quickly.
Halil:
- Yes, Captain.
- Do you hear a voice?
Halil:
- No, sir ...
- I guess you're too tired, you did not sleep a few nights Sir..
Ekrem:
- It might be ...you are done guys?
Halil:
- Captain, I have a few more jobs, and then we can go out ...
Ekrem:
- Okay, look at your job..
Halil:
-Yes, sir ..
Rahchan:

- Hey .. I'm here ..

Ekrem:

- Huh?

Rahchan:

- Look at the wall ...

Ekrem:

-I do not see it.but i hear.

Rahchan:

-Now look...

- I am Rahchan ..do you see...?

Ekrem:

- I saw it. Who are you now?

Rahchan:

- Fikret's ex-wife ...

Ekrem:

-How so....

Halil:

- We can go , Sir...

Rahchan:

- Shh ... Then we talk.

Ekrem:

- Halil you go..I'm coming in.

I think I've started to go crazy. I have heard self-gesticulating voices and started to see hallucinations. What kind of house is this? What kind of place ... In two minutes, all my psychology is down.

Rahchan:

- Do you hear me? Do not leave me alone here!

Ekrem:

- What?

Rahchan:

- Do not go ...

Ekrem:

- Come on, guys, shut up everywhere.

Halil:

- Ok Sir

After he handed over the work to the crew, the Captain kept his your house way for rest.

Ekrem:

- What was that? Was it really a hallucination? The deceased was also a strange person, and the house he lived in was never normal.

- Rahchan!

-Their neighbours never mentioned this name. They did not even say it was his wife.

-I've begun to lose my health, I guess. I should go to my psychologist Cansu tomorrow.

- I'm going to go back to that house again.

The commissioner fell into a deep sleep. In his dream, he began to see strange things again. He fell in love with some woman and left his job for this woman. He said that I would be a writer and I would stay with you.

Rahchan:

- Ekrem, come on.

-I'm waiting for you, come back ...

Ekrem:

- I do not even know you, Rahchan. Where should I come?

Rahchan:

-Come on, come on, come on ...

Ekrem:

-Oh my God , what kind of dream is this?

-Alo, Cansu ..

Cansu:

-Yes Ekrem, are you okay?

Ekrem:

- I'm not good.

Cansu:

-What happened? ..

Ekrem:

- I do not know.

-When i can see you?

Cansu:

- One second: Let's meet with you in another place.

Ekrem:

-Oh ... But my stomach is hungry, Cansu.

Cansu:

- I can buy you some..

Ekrem:

-No, is there a place you can eat without using any money?

Cansu:

-Why ?

Ekrem:

-Is there ?

Cansu:

- I have.

Ekrem:

- Let's go there then.

Cansu:

- But we need to car..

Ekrem:

- Car?

-Far ..?

-How far is Cansu ..?

Cansu:

-15 km.

Ekrem:

-Can we go there without using those metal piles and without using the money?

-What will happen, on foot ...

Cansu:

- Let's take a walk.

-Finally, come on in front of the Firuzaga Mosque in half an hour.

Ekrem:

-Good.

Ekrem:

-I've been waiting for you for fifteen minutes.Where have you been?

Cansu:

-I came here.

Ekrem:

-Where are we going?

Cansu:

-Balat ... Come on I'll take you to the my aunt ... she cooks for us now ...She will ready to meet us soon..We can speak on the road

- Tell me what's happening with you?

Ekrem:

-Cansu, we entered a house yesterday for a death sentence. A old man passed away silently.

-But..

Cansu:

-But?

Ekrem:

- I wanted to see you the house where my man lived. there was a lot of painting in each corner ..strange. The walls of the house was strange and all the walls are covered with articles and symbols. Anyway we were doing our case study in our own way. I also started to check the rooms one by one. I came across a lot of quirks and pictures that were written on the wall in the last room and were not read correctly.I began read to articles ,then started to hear some voices. So someone started to talk to me there.I was nervous at first. I said "i m going be crazy". I called Halil. He said he did not hear anything. I started to hear voices again. I said to myself that I am not sleeping for two days, so I started to see hallucinations. Somebody talked with me until I left the house. It came as I saw someone. What do you think?

Cansu:

-You've seen hallucination ... Ekrem .. not such a thing ... You lost a little awareness of extreme stress and skepticism because of your profession, and you have met with delusions. Now will go to my aunt place, and then I will give you a short therapy. .Do not worry..

Ekrem:

- Is that it?

Cansu:

-So ... Relax, leave yourself to me .. Do not stress.

Ekrem:

-OK..

After a long journey, Cansu and Ekrem came to the house of Cansu's aunt in Balat. The aunt prepared a table of classical home dishes. Ekrem followed Cansu's every moment until she had finished eating. Cansu was aware of this. It was impossible to not aware see Fikret emotions..

Ekrem:

-How interesting a woman that I have not noticed before?

-She was so repulsive when I was a student years ago ... I had other girls in my life.Maybe cos of i couldnt see that..

Cansu:

-Erkrem ...

-Yeah, come on, let's have a cup of tea here and then we can get you out of your worries.

-There is a balcony in the room, we can sit there, then you lie there and we apply something to you ..

Ekrem:

- It's okay.

Cansu:

-Ekrem ..

Ekrem:

-What?

Cansu:

-I'd like to admit that I found you more handsome than your old times.

Ekrem:

-Thank you .. I find you very beautiful.

Cansu:

-Thank you dear..

Ekrem:

-She said so sincerely! I liked..

- Cansu, tell me how you will treat this ...explain me plz..

Cansu:

-I will give you a treatment through hypnosis and I will remove the worries and suspicions in the head.

Ekrem:

- Will you do it? How?

Cansu:

-I will send some codes to certain parts of the brain with biomagnetic energy so that these thoughts are erased from the mind

-Relax and leave it to me...

Ekrem:

-OK...

Cansu:

- I have something ready, , and I want from you to be relax and concentrate on the music , and a kind of sleeping.

-You'll be back in forty-five minutes..I'm thinking of applying it a few more times ...

Ekrem:

- Let's do it ...

Cansu:

-Ekrem, do not look at me like that!

Ekrem:

- How do I look?

-I do not ...

Cansu:

-Come on, come on up here reach

CURE

Cansu played the set-musical, set was that Cansu could hypnotize to Ekrem easily, and he slept. he had been influenced by a deep hypnosis after five or six minutes ...

Rahchan:
-Hey Ekrem ...
-Do you hear me..?
Ekrem:
-Who are you?

Rahchan:
-Its Rahchan..look at me..
- I'm waiting for you now ...
-Do you hear?
Ekrem:
-I am hear you..
-Where did you find me..
Rahchan:
- It is very easy for me to find you Ekrem ..
-Let's get up .. You're so good .. There's nothing .. I'm real and always I'll be with you ..
Ekrem:
-I will come today Rahchan ..Okay ..Wait me..

When Ekrem awake, Cansu was watching him.

Cansu:

- Who's the Rahchan?

Ekrem:

-Rahchan? How do you know?

Cansu:

-You were talking to someone who was a Rahchan in hypnosis.

Ekrem:

-Yeah, I remember ... That's the person I heard her voice ...

Cansu:

- Ekrem should treat you seriously.

-Why ? You've started showing some serious disease symptoms.

Ekrem:

-No Cansu .. I'm fine ..

Cansu:

-You are good.Yes,Ekrem..good..

Ekrem:

-What? Yeah..

Cansu:

-I want to send you to another doctor ...

Ekrem:

-No, Cansu, I do not want to talk to anyone else ...

Cansu:

-Why Ekrem?

Ekrem:

-I said I do not want to.

Cansu:

-It's okay.I will help you..
Ekrem:
- I have to go now to Cansu.
Cansu:
-Where are you going?
Ekrem:
- I have to go.
Cansu:
- Then come back to my office in a few days, okay?
Ekrem:
-Okay Cansu ... I will be coming to you soon.

Cansu:
-Let you relax, Ekrem, I think it's temporary.
Ekrem:
- What, Cansu?
Cansu:
-This is what you've been through.
Ekrem:
- I hope so, too.So i am good..
-See you, Cansu.I love you..
Cansu:
-See you...

Ekrem left from Balat and started to drive to the house in Nişantaşı where he heard the voice of Rahchan.

-What are you doing, Ekrem?

-Do you really go crazy?

-You're so impressed with Rahchan, yes.

-I cant forget her face..I do not know if it was real or not ... but attracted to me .. I need to go there .. I want to see her again .. I hear her voice everywhere .. How a womans voice ..

-And if I could not hear it again, see her image again..it was real?

-She says that she is real...

-Are you real Rahchan?

-She was his wife? How it can be?

- How could it be like that?

-There's a voice, there is a figure but its like metaphysical thing

-Why is this Ekrem ...? Are you crazy?

- Is that what Cansu doing with this ?

Ekrem came to the apartment in Nişantaşı and silently walked into the apartment and after the seal on the door broke off, he opened the door with the credit card he had taken out of his pocket and went in. Without looking to his right or left, he sat in the seat in front of the window in front of the saloon and started to dive on the opposite wall looking at a violin paintings- ...

Ekrem:

-Why did he draw two eyes in the middle of something like this violin, a big night behind it, this violin like talking ... How can such strange things come out of a human being? I cant understand... There are hundreds of them on these walls.

Rahchan:

-Hey ..

Ekrem:

- What?

Rahchan:

-Yeah, here I am, look at your back.

Ekrem:

-Rahchan?

-You look so beautiful and you look young.

Rahchan:

- Thanks, Ekrem ..

-Thank you for coming.

Ekrem:

-You were calling me all the time and I came.

Rahchan:

- Yes, I did.

Ekrem:

- I can not understand what this thing is.

Rahchan:

-Do not you think of that Ekrem..you can see me?

Ekrem:

-Yeah..

-Please live me now..

Ekrem:

-Who would not want to live a beautiful woman like you?

Rahchan:

-Come here I want to kiss you Ekrem .. I'm very lonely ..I'm good you came .. Help me to relieve the pain ..

Ekrem:

-I will help you Rahchan..

Rahchan:

-Thank you..

Rahchan:

-You're not going to leave me, are you?

Ekrem:

-Yes, I will never let you go.

Rahchan:

-Please stay here with me all the time, please.

Ekrem:

-I can not stay here. We should go to my house..

Rahchan:

- Let's go, Ekrem ...

That night, Ekrem and Rahchan went to Ekrem's house. Ekrem had already fallen in love with that magical beauty of Rahchan. There was something in this woman that he would never give up on his mind. She actually feels good. It was true or not..He already did not think about it..The next morning, actually, he got up late at noon, handed over the letter of resignation, and began to live with the Rahchan in his new world. He deeply dived through the windows of the Bosphorus at night

CURE

and began to write to Rahchan in the darkness, but not to Rahchan..It was to Cansu..

DELUSION

Ekrem:
- And the other thing that is caught in my mind is the part of isolating yourself .. You can also save yourself from it .. you will be comfortable ..already everything flowing.. you have to be able to read this - Major - ..
- Do not stress to others life
- Its too hard..
- It makes you down
- Some people really suck energy
- I hope it helps.

- vimeo.com/91321071
- Let's see the promotional film we made.

- Are you in Nisantasi?
- I will come to you immediately and will give you this book -Major-

CURE

-?

- You have not sent your shoe's photo
- I'm starting the new book: name: Stiletto - will be k k

- I had an panic attack.

Ekrem:
- But there was excessive stress.
- Meanwhile, I am setting up another design workshop called major design
-Could this panic attack be of cosmic energies?
- Coca cola should not drink @
- :)

- www.majortasarim.com
- How did you find this site?
- Pardon
- I've sent the wrong
- http://www.majortasarim.net
- It
- We can work art here
- I made my speacial web last night
Rahchan:
-Let's write xanax to you

CURE

- There is
- A box.
- Have you looked at the site
- In the night i will take half xanax ...
- :)
- I did fight with 3 men ..
- I won..
- :)
 - In the clothes shop
 - I can give you a book...You could not read that somehow..

 Rahchan:
 -I did not like shoes
 Ekrem:
- Yours was very good.
- You did not sent me picture :)
- That would be the leg length.
- But shoot from the top
- This shoe's color and base design is very childish
 Rahchan:
-Cheap
 Ekrem:
- Yea

CURE

- The heel is very important.
- :)
- Stiletto

Rahchan:

-Nail polish is bad

-Giuseppe Zanotti makes good

-Anyway ...

Rahchan:

- :) Italy
- Okay
- Sexy gold
- After that I will make secret photo shoots .
- It was not the photo I had in mind ... But shooting should be in your work room and I missed that..But we destroyed to inspirations..
- Inspiration
- Nail Polish sounded a nice word,
- Make a painting with nail polish

Ekrem:

- Well, welbutrin has begun to sell again here
- Zanotti sells his shooes min. 600$
- What do you think creative direction or art direction for me?

Ekrem:

- Something like paranormal sexuality, which may be between metaphysical and physical, comes to mind.When i say that :son of God

- Why there's no daughter of God.

Rahchan :

-The devil has a daughter.

- Satan is not God.

Ekrem:

- Who is the devil's daughter? It's paranormal to be a daughter of Satan ... Who is the daughter of the devil?

- If the devil has a daughter, it means no difference from us.

- How do I look at you?

- My shadow is speaking :

- The novel is starting late in the night

- Is it? :)

- Do you need design a card viz?

- I've seen Aslı and Funda in the night

-Look at Photo

- What do you think ,is she.. Aslı ..50 years old?

- How do you interpret:How a cat recognise to fish as food?

-Plz..look at this photo too..
- This baby is 8 years old
- In Marmaris
- He needs Marrow transplant
- Unowned
- Make donation for him
- I want to be assisted him and wait for your help.

Ekrem:
- He yo
- How are you?
- Tell me about the devil's daughter :)
- A very interesting question: What is the first image that comes to your mind from the time you come to the world and your the old one memories..and how old was
- I remember even some dreams I saw at 4 years old
- You should always keep hungry
- Very toughness is not good.
- Who always keeps hungry can be open minded
- People makes always wrong in toughness
 Rahchan:
-I remember when i was 3-4 old ..

CURE

Ekrem:

- Well then
- :)
- Your Alzeimer risk very low
- I wanna ask something
- Women's psychology
- I went to the business appointment yesterday ,one company invited me for art management..
- A girl investigated me..and called..
- Anyway
- I went to business negotiations to there
- The girl told me the whole life of her
- She got Leukemia before then survived
- And she learned that i am tao and quantum yogo trainer
- She talked about them outside of work during interview
- I'm thinking..
- So why did she call me!
- Is it such a job interview?
- And spoke of An information sharing center on me
- I said I am an artist, but I can improve you in a biomagnetic environment
- I tired to walk until Galata..

Rahchan :

- Strange ..

Ekrem:

- Yeah Weird

CURE

Rahchan:

- Result?

Ekrem:

- It's strange to tell some when you met at the first time of all special life

Rahchan :

-It can be

-She tought that you are Guru

Ekrem:

- Interesting that , I'm focused on the cancer of the blood for 2-3 days

Rahchan:

-You get job?

Ekrem:

- Could be

-We did not speak of job ! I wonder that she will back or not!

- I told her about surreal minimalism, psychedelic art

- She only looked at me..

Rahchan :

-Maybe meet you?

-Whether she is setting?

-Let's see

Ekrem:

- So!

- I guess..

- Nice girl too..

- I will send you her photo..

- Do you need something from me?
- Look
- This girl

Rahchan:
- Yeah..
- Beautiful

Ekrem:
- Yes i liked her too
- I love blonde..
- If I will doing Setting then
- It would be bad for her.
- I'll bring you the -major- in this times, I've sent it to the some Japanese.

Rahchan:
- Ekrem there is some one who: Can convert to my draw to a professional architectural style?

Ekrem:
- There is

Rahchan :
-You?

Ekrem:
- I can try it..Send me your file to me..
  - I can use Sketchup..

Rahchan:
- You know this is an architect doing it.
-It's not the Picture

CURE

Ekrem:
- What did you draw? Is it for inside or outside?
Rahchan:
- I thought about something once for a place
- I actually took the architect with me.
- But his head is very slow..
- He should think, and think about on..
Ekrem:
- I have some masters of that
- I can take care of it.
- What we will do? How?
Rahchan:
- They should draw about what I think..
Ekrem:
- You want something 3D?
- What's the scenario?
Rahchan:
- No need for now
Ekrem:
- I will try for you..
Rahchan:
- Its Settling in a bay
Ekrem:
- Free
- To you :)
- Reference for me..
- My composition..
- I have no diplomas just

Rahchan:
-Who has diploma makes procrastination to deal..
Ekrem:
- Is there something futuristic in the head?

Rahchan:
- It is in the Gocek.
Ekrem:
- OK..
Rahchan:
-No
-I wanna design ancient something
- It's never modern..
Ekrem:
- Let's make an antique structure.
Rahchan :
-Do you have your staff?
- Mezoroman style
- Lykia.
Ekrem:
- Yes i have staff..
- Yes
- Lycia discovery of money
- This will be built by engineers
- I will do it based on her
- How many square feet of land?
- Do you have maps?
Rahchan:

CURE

- I will tell you

-What do you think ..i should take architect?

-I think so they are bullshit!

Ekrem:

- Let's write the script..

- Let's give it to a crazy talented psycho architext, who needs money

Rahchan:

-Lets meet now with you?

Ekrem:

- Ok When do you want meet me?

Rahchan:

- Who is this psycho?

Ekrem:

- There is a madman in the city of Ankara..

- :)

 Rahchan :

-You know ,i do not have time.

Ekrem:

- I am in charge for you..Ok?

- I will create the golden bay for you..

- Again

Rahchan :

-They said:

-Could be your dreams

-Should nobody intervenes to you

-Etc.

-Etc.

CURE

Ekrem:
-Okey, let's look at it together.
- Then we will create your dream world..
- By talking

Rahchan :
-Can you help me?
Ekrem:
- I do..
- Willingly
- I love you so much..
Rahchan:
- Come to my place today!
Ekrem:
- Okay
- When?
Rahchan :
- To Forest houses
Ekrem:
- OK
Rahchan:
-Is it far?
Ekrem:
- I do not know
Rahchan:
- Or meet tomorrow in the center?
Ekrem:
-How you want..where you relax..

- I will design..

Rahchan:

-I am here today

-But I have to get it

-And I am impatient

Ekrem:

- This place near by a Lake?

- Is it very far away

Rahchan:

- Yes

Ekrem:

- Send me direction

Rahchan :

-40 min

Ekrem:

- Get there by public transportation ?

- :)

- If there is no car..difficult

Rahchan:

-Tomorrow we can meet..

Ekrem:

- I have to rent a car

- Good for tomorrow morning

Rahchan:

-10 am?

Ekrem:

- Okay, deal

- Ok

- I have two gifts for you, one for the -major- and one 75!
   - See ya.
Rahchan:
- Thank you

Ekrem:
- No problem

Ekrem:
- If you think that I will make your entitlement as well :)
- The architect is okay.
Rahchan:
- Something strange happened to these stone houses, I say tomorrow is a really strange idea
 Ekrem:
 - There is a problem with putting
-You need to solve it once
Rahchan:
-It's a very difficult legal process.
-Now is not right to do something
-Meaningless
- I do not know
-My morale is so bad.
Ekrem:
- Wow
- No problem
- Whenever possible

- But there's a terrific idea.
- I will dissolve it in the state :))
- Reaching the day
- With the State
- We will solve..
- Is the problem reconstruction?
- Is it the Council of State?
- if this works out, I'm hooking up with a crazy organization.

Rahchan:

-Where did it come from?

-I do not know

-Very hot yet

- Ok we can help

Ekrem:

- Keep in your mind
- Be relax-
- It's always this way
- I have an acquaintance.
- Even my father will solve those issues if it is not very deeply fielded
- I was excited :)
- Anyway
- Rahchan

Rahchan:

-Think of me

Ekrem:

- Yes

- I lost job of 150 carat royal emerald before
- I understand
- Even dreaming was beautiful.
- I created opportunities from this crisis.
- I agreed with some partners for architeact business
- I'm going to try this idea in Alacatı..
- I will show you when done
- Of course my idea is to design to those stone homes
- Actually I created a business line..
- Life is very creative :) you do not worry.
- I say it from my heart..

- Look at the crazy thing.
- Let's do a painting with you
- Get ready
- :)
- Creative director is you are
- And let's do it
- Let's make a model of in mind.
- Lets buy materials
- Stationery
- And let's make model

Rahchan:
-I want to do the my Bay.

Ekrem:
- :)
- We will make a model for that
- When it will finish..the problem of Bay will solved

CURE

- That Ankara society
- There is Demir Construction
- His son is my childhood friend
- I told them that
- They said ok.
- So we do not see you tomorrow then?
- I want to be a life coach

Rahchan:

-I would like to see you.

Ekrem:

-Let me do the model

-I can go to deputy for problem solve ..

Ekrem:

-That brain surgeon should know what he cuts off.
- The man said america.
- Why do not we do it?
- I think I will settle for a while around New York
- One last thing: do you believe evil eye? I took this to bad energy..then felt too weak myself... the way is clear ..ah these women are so dangerous.. ..

Rahchan:

-I made an evil eye?

Ekrem:

- No

- You got it
- You have found the evil eye.
- It might be a little ahead.
- Like magic
- My tobacco is pure nicotine :)
- Result: i distroyed to this fucken woman around you ..

Rahchan:

- -Major- you can do to me
-Best gift
-I am reading now..

Ekrem:

- Please read it.
- Major has been coded hardly by me..Can be there some spelling errors.
- I bumped the power of that woman..

Rahchan:

- It's full of Assosiations. Foam!
-Immovable
-Mysterious
-Wise
-Clever
-Brave and innovative
-I work on it
-Should Precise print
-About me
-But i asked myself that cos of i impressed from this..
 - But I am induce to speak to you
--I am invisible but I am in

-It must be a film
-Correspondence screen 16: 4
-Covered
-And it should be just speech
-Just hear keystrokes
-Message came..

-Other Stages
-in the Street
-At hospital
-Etc

Ekrem:
- Yesss
- Senarotif..
- You finished Immediately
- Super

Rahchan:
- Should Structured
-Let's do

Ekrem:
- Let's do this lucky work.

Rahchan:
-There is a movie Jude Law in and Julia Roberts
-Watch how it start
-A correspondence screen

Ekrem:
- I know that film
- It must be a schizoid screen

- So the screen will be designed again under the transparent screen

Rahchan:

-Enough for the first 5 minutes.

- Watch ..after boring

- Just a purist correspondence

-The content

-Already strong

-No need for anything

- They can not understand

Ekrem:

- High..

- Do not break concentration

- I told you the name of my new book

- Do you remember a night when I took to a photo at 4 am of the night

- Name: My Shadow is Talking

Rahchan:

-Yeah.

Ekrem:

- I will solve the -major- problem now

- I have seen you and I have given you evil.

- Only you know of My Shadow is Talking

- Just you

- You do not appear but like you are

- :) My shadow is talking

Rahchan:

-Yeah

-I will read it too

-But neuroscience is good topic

-Populer happens

Ekrem:

- Is it?

- Okay, let's work out the -Major- with you..Ok?

- Psycho topic

- Let's work

Rahchan:

-Interesting

-I will show an to writer..

Ekrem:

- Okay thank so much.

- I wonder what he says

- Neuroscience is an elite ... I wonder now

Rahchan:

- I need more neutral critic

- A critical

-But I am right

-This high-level dissociation is good..

-Its shots Zeitgeist from his heart

-And it is crushing

Ekrem:

- He he

- Yess

- And open-minded

- Apart from that, metaphysics also puts points

Rahchan:

-Last sentence

Ekrem:

-For the book would be the best interpretation

- Thanks a lot

- What I noticed is that on you.. You have a noble heart

- Thank you

- I will help you of your problems

- And you will help me with - major-.

- Let's make a movie

Rahchan:

- I sure do.

Rahchan:

-I already wanted to and I was dreaming write of a neuroscience one day

-I could not write the book ..

-But the examples

-It came very dry

-How to make..

-This is very clean-cut

-You should write..

Ekrem:

- I'm super excited

- If you let me, I will make an application to you someday of biomagnetic..

CURE

Rahchan:
- I will call your father again for the bay
- I want that Mert will tell him something again
- I do not want to any problem there

Ekrem:
- OK
- I said to my father that you will call again..

- It must be all right today
- Mert talked with ours
- My dad called now me..
- You can be relax.
- He has some deputy friends..
- Do not worry now..
- We talked.

Rahchan:
-Okay thank you,Ekrem..

Ekrem:
- We will do to Bay
- We can host them someday
- Then everything will be ok..

Rahchan :
-OK

Ekrem:
-I have no necktie

Rahchan:

- Ok i will buy for you..

Ekrem:

- Do not worry these undergrounds problems

- Yes i want necktie

Rahchan:

-Underground ??

-I do not understand exactly

Ekrem:

- We can talk then..

- A kind of gang is infected to you ..I think so..

- I was feeling

- So..your husband did not tell you

- You will not open this to him..

Rahchan:

-I will call you Ekrem

-If you want after 1 hour

Ekrem:

- Ok

- Call.

-I swear to God I want to help you more now

- :)

- By the way, I watched the film - Closer- Julia and Jude played that you mentioned, I've seen it again before, there is a mistake of the writer character there. In these usa-made films, they always explain the same mistake.

- http://m.imdb.com/title/tt0120601/

- Did you watch this?

CURE

Ekrem:

- Did you wake up

- Look at the model

Rahchan:

-Did you do that?

Ekrem:

- Yea

Rahchan:

Ekrem:

-You are amazing

- I'm working on a little bit

- Do not worry.

- I guess that's right for you.

  - The top side entrance to pier

- Anything else? I can come to hospital and join to operation :))

- Now only need make your construction

- And now tell me about setup in your mind of me

- I worked on for 9-10 hours in the night

- I wont much more

- I will give you that

- We can add attachments or something

- I'm really tired.
- I read the user guide in 2 hours
- This is
- I think the architect who would put his head on and think about sleeping would give it to you in 2- 3 months or so,
- There's a courtyard there.
- The stone worker can do something with as Turkish style
- There is restaurant part and a place extra cafe-restaurant..others can be shop
- The oven can be in the restaurant
- There is also a place can workshop for production..
- Apart from that there is a room for the staff,I also have small rooms for guests'
- The place at the front of the road ,Suitable for all kinds of needs
- There is all kinds of parking around there
- Can made up of many different toilet areas
- energy part electric gas etc. whatever it is infrastructure construction
- Or you need to know what infrastructure is there
- I made the pool the depth of the pool etc.. what you decide or can remove
- But the pool can be any kind of bar around it
- You can do the occasional wedding there
- So there's the capacity to make an event ...
- You can sunbathe

- It must already be a market.

- There is a long way

- Archway, can also be made in certain parts of flowered archway

- Look now..its your antique stone avm :)

- The entrance section for orange and mandarin cologne, jam cherries etc etc etc ..

- Production can done there as well

Rahchan :

-Thank you

-Design is exactly your job

- I am an office statement

-I will work for my project at this night

Ekrem:

- You'r welcome..i created this from your mind..

- It may be simpler or more simple, but it can be basic to project sub-structure

- I designed something for the courtyard to be built in.

- If it goes, there will be a bigger courtyard.

- The building which cuts from the center is the extra entrance gate again with arched

- So you can tell these to person who gonna built this yard

Rahchan:

-I want Mardin architect

Ekrem:

-I can get it out of from there.. I just looked at them yesterday

- Mardin architecture is can on the project
- It's fantastic
- High ceiling arcs
- Stone houses 3000 years old they are original
- Under the lots of treasure
- Do you forget my book and sent it to the author?

Rahchan:

-Even I sent.

Ekrem:

- Super ...Thanks..
- You are crazy too :)
- This madness is the line between genius and mad
- I do not think there is only one thing in my book they will not like..
- And it's finishing like going to continue anyway
- After we can check other my books..
- For write to this book ,i read more than 30 books,traveled 6 countries and internet works..we should not underestimate to internet..I told you before of Tor.
- I pay attention to your estimate more than Literature
- The result of that you are scientist
- Not a writer
- You need to know that how Schopenhauer is talking to the literary drama :(
- The last phone speech we spoke today brought a very crazy scenario to my mind for the next of major ..Metaphysical detective

CURE

- Part 2 is My shadow is talking
- If were a film ,Nejat should play in this
- You more elegant ..Like you people should read that..

Ekrem:

-Heyo
- I found a girl
- Guess her profession
- I dont want to show my creatings to these roughs..my avant-garde status starts from where i starting to think that they can not think..

- Do you have an account in the abroad?
- For the sale of these books..
- A Cubist ,Pakistani and Jew
- What a strange world :)
- Cyprus is a beautiful island ..These islands
- Oh these islands
- Look
- Opened the whole world with this process
  - We will not underestimate what the Internet is.
- :)

- Rahchan
- 3 bottles of whiskey arrived
- You will take it ? From Italy..

- For three bottles he says 500 tl..
- Original
- Cheap

Rahchan:

-I do not know ..I have never buy Whiskey

Ekrem:

- Buy for your man
- Ask him
- Drink whiskey for good men
- I bought one..I drink rarely
- I'm in Cihangir. This is cihangir trip..
- There is everything
- Rahşaann what do you think my life is crazy..or yours?
- :)
- Do not hike with me..
- I found a girl
- Architect
- Look at the picture.
- This girl..Her name is Ahu
- How?

Rahchan:

-Cool

Ekrem:

- Yea
- We will meet tomorrow
- What do you think where she lives?

-)

- Topağacı

- Nishantshi..

- The power of little things

- Much stronger

- A voice from my inside says that we will not be able to be in touch for a while .. I would like to see you when I made a correspondence with Mor .. but I am silent ..

- Bye

 Rahchan:

-Mor also wrote to me.

Ekrem:

- In times she is in a jam

- Now look:

- I do not know ..i live 30 square meters place in Gümüşsuyu..Pay for that 1000 tl

- She pays 5000 tl for her flat..and spends a lot of money..

- I'm eat pasta ..she eats chop

 Rahchan:

-You're right.

Ekrem:

- Who is in poor?

- I do not feel sorry for her

- She was always tricky..

- I have good friends..its enough for me..
- I tell you
- I dont care about her..

Rahchan:

-Ekrem

-I did not write to you because you be sorry for her.

-I'm tired of listening to her

-Because I dont live her life..

-I work as a civil servant ..and its my life style

Ekrem:

- Yes I told you to delete her from your life ..
  - Delete her
- You will be very comfortable

Rahchan:

-And I always stay helpless when we speak with her

-My head today swollen

Ekrem:

- Do not listen her
- Look, I'm friendly to you
- True friend
- Friend
- I know you.
- If you believe me..

Rahchan :

- I understand

Ekrem:

- Delete her .. block her ..dont listen her..
- You will pray to me..

CURE

-There are so less jobs in this world that I can not finish..

- I dont ever expected anything from you.

Rahchan:

- Are you okay

-Ekrem?

Ekrem:

- You are my friend..

-I am very well today

- High energy

Rahchan:

-Be good

-Please

- Did you feel a bad thing?

Ekrem:

- Your feeling is normal: I gave up Efexor and started to Xanax

- :) original

- Think of your own dreams..

Ekrem:

- I have to live things to complete my book..

- I experienced part of that ..for development part approx i need more

- I will become a famous writer and will live my works after me..

- Others lie..

- A person who does not have any humor who can not make a joke, even her smile is a fake, and who is always telling trouble, does not do anything without sucking energy.

- There was a guy , I wanted to help him on a very good job, I found a good channel for him first: owner to told me that the ask your friend: there is 8-year-old child who is leukemia ... and send for him money how you can ... I called and said him this .. but he did not help to kid..the name of the company i dont say you now..then company owner did not give him this big job.

- Same thing: he is ..this guy ..for another job too made like that and lost again a big job..

- Look ..now my books are in Japan..

- No longer

- Do you understand of cosmetics?

- Sometimes what i think you know, like generally being in the world really forbiden for me..

- Because nothing in the world has really excited me

- Study, women, nature, people ... you have to eat food or something like that, and Sometimes i feel hungry sometimes not hungry..

- Fat and sugar

CURE

- One girl called in the morning.
- Good morning ..how are you..
- Bla bla..
- She said I'm close to you
- I said come over and i will make some coffee.
- You come on, I said invitations
- She said :no, i invite to you something eat..
- Then she said that :i m a virgin.
- She said,i learned to kissing from a girl..
- Then she paid to bill..
- After that i gave to her my expensive ring..
- Anyway
- I did not like that she paid that..
- I said ok..in the evening when you finish your jobs come to me and we can kissing
- Actually, I do not even have a kiss with this girl.
- She seeking a experience
- Mor called and said that we are close friends
- Rahchan,You got me excited twice.
- Blow it again ..
- I changed your name in the my phone book ..now your are someone else
- You are now,Arben!

- I need to see you
- Are you around here today?
- Do you write me xanax?

- To jealous,love games .. affectation..etc.etc. set up on set up, bed games ,love games in the bed..couldnt deceive..
- I need the girl with the brains :)
- She came tonight
- We saw that she was not a virgin.
- At the moment i have 3 women
- 2 turkish and 1 russian
- The Russian married and she cheating her husband with me.. anyway its normal for her..
- One of the Turkish is without me sleeps with others too..
- 3rd seeking rich husband ..
- I will busy 7 days a week
- When i changed your name, you have completely lost the effect on me
- Rahchan = a big zero ,now
- The real Rahchan now zero, Rahchan in the -major- never spoke with me ..Arben came and cleaned you from my mind..
- I will not write you anymore.
- Arben there must be a relief inside of you today
- Arben, you were know that I wrote this -Major- in five months, not in a day.
Why it was seem to you like one day ?
-Sometimes you can feel it yea?
- Can you make my portrait?
- With my bow tie and jacket!

- I will wearing glasses

- It will be a book cover

- I want a portrait like a Shopen

- Like this..

- I do not think you're an artist. You have a lot of mistakes.

- :) Arben came and made great me..

- I said to Mor that i changed to my therapist..

- I m going soon from here..

- Thank you for your invitations

- The story was a lot of fun with you

- I do not know the Mert , but one day we will meet together..

- Thanks for your help..

- I made a big monology experience on this.

- The last gift

- When I was talking to you, I discovered something different in the process, knowing or not knowing .. I say myself :punish someone of that.. or what Simone said?

- Rahchan,Your diagnosis is not true of my bipolar semptoms

- I will go to another doctor..

- I will go

- He does not know all my business

- I tell you something about me ..tell him different

- Rahchan :

-Ekrem

-Daddy called me

CURE

-I understood, okey

Ekrem:

- Do not interference
- ok..
- I do not tell him everything
- I write to you, always a monology fiction.
  - You see, I'm right.
- Hippocratic oath !
- You are from my family and my friend
- I'm always in the back of you..
- I should have seen that my Shadow is talked..
- Hard to detect me
- I'm sensing you.No problem..
- And everybody talked of me.
- Was I that shade?
- My father talked and he talked about me..
- You talked..and you talked about me..

-Everyone talked about me but I was not there..
- Who was he?
- My shadow!
- Strong Design ! Literature can not understand these
- Someone should notice this ability
- Then literature will notice to new trend's pioneer
- Destiny,may be after a long time.
- Do not make me an officer in the work life and do not lock up me
- I can escape again.

CURE

- I call my own trend - Subliminalism -

- Does your art need this innovation? Yes..all needs that..

- You were all authority and you are so motivated ... I have weakened your authority by directing all of you .. I told you that I have done this .. I have programmed your system .. I have tried to hack your brains .. have you been an authority or have you programmed as authoritarian System? .. it should have been programmed different for everyone then they were lived like human..

- You should be shock from this words now ,as a scientist

- Art is a science too.

- You said to my dad that you will call me at 7 pm

Rahchan:

- I will call

-I am now on my way

Ekrem:

- Ok.

- https://en.m.wikipedia.org/wiki/Methaqualone

- Rahchan, Do you give to this lithium ? If you you must know that what you give up lithium you can live really bad trips.. I think you must give her Efexor..

- The fall of lithium is painful

- Can you hypnotize the patient and put him in the trans ...?

- Lithium is bad ... can make kidney problems.

- It's my opinion

- https://youtu.be/ZIxyPkeAyDc

- You too love sarcasm ...I saw that ..

- :)

- Lithium stay in blood... when the woman got pregnant, lithium can pass to baby like virus..

- Look at this?And think about it..

- Baby can be Epileptic ..

- I found the way to shoot out from blood, but i do not say it;)

- Thinking about the reason why lithium is staying in: lithium metal is a noble element ... there is a lithium in body ..if you add more ,maybe you can create a new magnetic process in the body ..its good for brain..?...could be hard shoot out them from body?

- https://youtu.be/g8ecLZtPssQ

- Final track

- ok..

- Look at the man's age and energy

- I'm like this guy

- Comment ?

- 3 years ago. I have been subjected to the invitible organization of 4 women ..That time I have taken in my mind paxil seroquel .They have met me a girl .. I understood that this devil's daughter is indeed the devil's daughter ... I walked around with her on the London's sidewalks ... The her mother and the other women were psychologically attacked to my cancer father ... she traveled with Ekrem ...and she tought that he is too incapable.. We returned to home..then she wanted to London again... What i did to this: i went to London with her ... We traveled again in the streets.. ... i said the money finished .. We wandered around the streets with suitcases for a whole day ..in the night we sat in the seats behind a apartment ... She stayed on the street ... i saw her fear and helplessness..Then i watched with amazement the methods taught for exploitation that her family teach her..

- What happened?
- She is fled from fear..
- You can give me all drugs ..but i can solve all problems on this high mind
- What was the my intentions? ..First i really wanted to help to her of health and pecuniary
-Now ,I look at the chair behind that building..
- I'm looking
- :)
- at The Big Easy Kings Road, Chelsea
312-314 KINGS ROAD, London

- My team..
- Russian is more dangerous
- You remember people said about me that i m gay ,russian,jewish,drug dealer,crazy,mental etc etc
- Sometimes I can not understand who i am !

CURE

- I was a satanist too..:)..Before one man saw my books and said about me that i am satanist..But these books were about philosophy!

- In USA shamans started to work in hospital
- They are talking about the feature of self-fix and scan in the brain that I mentioned before..
- I was shocked when i saw that on TV!
- Alternative Medicine
- Placebo !!!
- Cerebellum
- Before i wrote you of that..
- Doctors now afraid of Shamans..
- Rahchan, those writers read to my book?
-?
- Just tell me where is the entrance door where I can send magnetic resonance to the brain..where is? .. Where can I send the code to the brain .. ?
- Did you hear
- Me?
- :)
- https://youtu.be/B8MZdu-g7vo

Ekrem:
- Is it black or white? Honey or strawberry?
- I got 4 certificates
- I can work as a psychologist now

- 2 from Russia

- For 15 days i was speaking with a girl..she told me all of her life..

- Today she said to me

- I do not correspond to people who i do not know

- :)

- He is me! That she doesnt know!

- She gave me before her mobile phone number..:),and now says like that..

- Rahchan

- I missed you..

- You are the most intelligent women I've ever met

- The real woman ..

- :)

- Can we clone you?

- That girl said that :I should be cool.

- I said fuck cool moods

Rahchan :

-What will you do with me?

Ekrem:

- I can not do something to you now

- If it can be before..

- Could be..

- I would always be beside you if i got you before..

- Those girls now..want to play games like kids..

- How do you design the dream you will see before you go to bed at night?

- I get a picture for dream scenario

- Before i jump into the rem
- Then you falling asleep whatching dream about the picture..

- I said to that girl:
- You're like a trucker when you're driving.
- Look at the arms.
- She was shock
- She wanted take revenge
- She can never do that!
- I will send you very cool set
- Listen
- https://youtu.be/a79xoHEesuA
- Listen to this set when you have time.
- I say do not read..i say listen :)
- I have more than EdMR..
- I can build a psycho-rehabilitation center with you.
- Here doctors using machine for magnetism
- But i use for this my hands
- CEREBELLUM!
- AND BROCA AREA
- I will work from here
- Major- seems like my thesis now

- Now if I come to you as a clinical psychologist and i will say you that i will work in a clinic, would you not be a reference with your wet signature for me?

- You will.

- As if Freud and Jung were very normal men in their heads?

- Look at the tattoo in the picture
- I will tell you what is that..
- I talk to you, and then Mor calls
- He yo
- I wont answer
- !
- ?
- I will not work with fake people.
- Sometimes I think that you look like her!
- Do you look like her?
- I love blond..She look like black grape..:)
- This is the situation
- You look a bit like her.
- I designed a model for you for 9 hours.Then you did not say Thank You..
- Then you do not even speak of that..
- But you said befor: let's do it together.
- Are there any similarities between you and the her?
- The Mor only can drink coffee with me and and can make a leg show, but a huge zero in qualification
- Her conversation not worth a cent
- She always send me promotion gifts
- starbucks.voucherpromotion.com
- Look at this!

CURE

- I miss always to Simone!
- Always i remember her
- Morcan make you bad things..be careful
- How many times have you disobey your hypocrite?
- You are so nebbish..cos you are friend with Mor
- Very sadly
- Wow
- I feel sorry for you
- Now
- I told all of my family that you still friend with her..
- You can not call anymore
- Father, very angry now
- It was good
- By
- :)

- You said to my father that I lied unconsciously
- I lied to you?
- Can you give me an example
- I need you to apologize to me for it.
- What lie?
- I did not say anything like that
- OK

- I have a lot of documents and diplomas I want to work as a psychologist
- Look at them, doctor.

CURE

- What do you think?

- Do i work?

Rahchan:

-It would be great.

- Beautiful

- I started to seek a new job

- Training is over

- Now I can work like an expert

Rahchan:

-Here you go..

Ekrem:

- I attended seminars:

- Quantum integration to psychology and neuro

- Osho

- Qigong ex

- Quantum yoga

Rahchan:

- I jealous you now

- I have all of them .. :) look you're a doctor

- I will apply to you something

- Allow me

- I m not doctor

- But we can be Agreed.

- You're a doctor, i m a master.

Rahchan:

-Maestro

Ekrem:

- Exactly

CURE

- I need to start in clinic..
- Now, think about what we can do together.

- I saw you again in my dreams..i saw you with Mert ..And i have saw one bespectacled boy ..You were coming to my uncles house in Istanbul..
-The first you were coming then Mert..And you met with all my family..Mert was swing Tasbih..
- Do you have abespectacled boy with the same type you?

Rahchan:
-Yeah

Ekrem:
- I saw his face my dream ..his face in front of my eyes now..
- Like age 7 -8 -9 or something
- He look like blond or auburn
- Then there was another girl who was older than him, taller than you, and they are said : hey mother ... mother ...we are here...and they came running in...
- It was a dream..
- That boy!
- My comment is that he is a very precious baby
- So i think like that
- It will be something.

Rahchan:
-What a beautiful thing you said

- Do not forget that!
- I saw it very clear
- He will be important something..
- Did you tell me about a lawyer girl?She is single?

Rahchan:

-Yeah

  -Single

- Do you have her picture
- Send me
- Of course,if she want..
- What do you think?
- I say constructive thought.
- Can try ?

Rahchan :

-There's someone else in her profile picture ....

-I have no her picture

- A :)
- What's her name?
- Do you want ,i can advise to you a book?
- Do you have a reading head?
- I will propose something.That girl..! I believe that i will see here anywhere..
- You can tell her that I want to see her picture
- I will do it
- OK
- Book: neuro-science: Artur Schopenhauer -Parerga ve Paralipomena - find this precisely ..
- It must be in D & R

CURE

Rahchan:

- ok..

Ekrem:

- Super book ..

Ekrem:

- Explosion

- Safe?

Rahchan:

- Yes

Ekrem:

- Ok..

- Rahchan,the person is can be so happy but it can not be too long..if there any unhappy people

- These people can suck energy

- :)

- I look after kindergartens to work

- What do you think.. job is the most basis baby and children

Rahchan :

CURE

- Could be
- Liberate them

Ekrem:
- Exactly the same..i will teach them to freedom
- They wont depressive grow up..
- By the way
- I developed a method for improve panic attack
- You have to see...

- 100% result
- I apply to this method and after 2 days in the night i got good result
- Application is good
- But 6 months before patient should come to you
- I call this the "sub-method"
- You have to see when the illness improve how body react to that..
- Do you wanna learn?

- I m starting work on Autism !
- I will make therapy to autistic kids
- *
- CEREBELLUM
- I said before..
- If they need a reference for this job , ai will give them your name and number?

CURE

- You can say them of me that he is a well-groomed clinical psychologist :)
- There's a terrific fascism explotion in the country.
- Look at the perception
- This battle signal.
- That Fırat Kalkanı
- The incident..
- Cos of we got attack in BJK
- Turkish war
- And will be winner in the Sout Syria
- Could be finish soon ..We are so tired..
- They asked me you were a psychiatrist?
- My dear colleague psychologists have listened to the autism neuroanatomy by me..
- They are very weak
- They love of salary and this dull them..
- They do not read books..
- It can be change..They must study more
- You did not take attantion of my sub procedure Rahchan..
- You did not take attantion to the major too, for read a my book i waited long time. I can teach you the method of your life
- But this time it's free.

Rahchan :

-OK

Ekrem:

- Ok..

- Its method really so strong..

- I can hypnotize you first and teach you what you need to do..

- You will have to put your patient the hospital and apply it for 1 hour.And will apply 5 times that

- Then patient come back after once a month

- First you will heal panic attacks

- Then social phobia

- I'm going to charge you for that and then you will improve all disorders

- Then!

- I can teach you things for autism, it's a long progress

- But it will really develop to all methods

- Create a system to work in the room

- I am telling you that the psychologist can make pedagogy in our land.

- This type therapy should be a psychiatrist job

- Psychiatrist

- So plus a group of patients will be added, psychologists should make pedagogy

- Sexual problems are even easier

- Rahchan:

-You should tell me more. Sometime

 -I will go to a lesson this weekend

- 1 week i m not here..

Ekrem:

CURE

- I will tell you practical narrative
- Very complex my system
- I make you a master

Rahchan:

-I understand

Ekrem:

- I made an application today.
- You can get result when patient sleeping
- This method is not something I've learned from anyone.. -I've developed.
- I come to teach you these ..
- Wait, comes another Rahchan

- WERNICKE
- Overcoming procrastination
- You have this problem too
- Why do you have this ?
- Leave the cigarette

Rahchan :

-Yes, I will quit

-What is procrastination ?

Ekrem:

- Its mean delay ,put off

Ekrem:

CURE

- Smoking takes your energy

Rahchan :

-Yeah

Ekrem:

-Interesting

-Word

- Important

  Rahchan :

  -Hey, there's a hypnosis method to give up smoke.

  - You can learn it.

- Easy

-:There is a place in Istanbul I want to go to these days.

Ekrem:

- Where?

Rahchan :

-Innercenter

- But the guys do not open their phones.

Ekrem:

- Why?

Rahchan :

-Maybe they abandoned to country.

Ekrem:

- Foreigners ??

- Who are they?

Rahchan :

-They were Hypno-Therapist

- And very successful.

Ekrem:

CURE

- I can win them
- Turkish man here..
- Rahchan
- Doctor.

  Rahchan :
- I did not go ,scared

Ekrem:
- My unluckiness is my type..my view is too grim
- My face and views too grim..its my nature :
- I can make you Hypnotize
- You can quit fast smoking
- You can heal your procrastination
- And treat the patients too

- We do it where you trust the most.
- In your hospital
- Hey Rahchan
- With bioenergy i can send codes to brain from magnetic area
- Hypno-Therapists can not know wernike
- I get done everything to brain.

Rahchan :
- I'm telling you
- To tell me about it

Ekrem:
- OK

CURE

- If I tell you and install to your brain and you do it automatically, easy
- When you are available,

Rahchan:

-Hocus pocus?

Ekrem:

- I need a sound system.
- Scientific lab
- No hocus mokus
- Scientific and pathological
- You take some drugs..i feel it..
- What is it in generally?

Rahchan :

-What ? I take

-Vitamins

-Flaxseed oil

-Cinnamon and curcuma

-The only thing harmful is the cigarette

-I will give up it

Ekrem:

- Leave the cinnamon too
- Vitamins are pills?

Rahchan :

-Yeah

Ekrem:

- Which is harmful to you?
- Can be B series
- Too much

CURE

- I wanna ask something
- Now I'm here in the clinic. How many money they want for quit smoking cigarettes therapy?

- How many hours do you sleep?
- I can help you for quit smoking while you were sleeping
- 8 hours
- Its takes 8 hours
- We can open with you outer center, doctor.
- Doctor we need a saloon + 2 rooms and 1 massage table
- your insider Semra is gone from Turkey
- :) in every condition we are here
- You make your last name SMITH ! :))
- Hehe
- I make without mashine to brain stimulation
- Today i spoke a lot..see you soon..

-;)
- 65% of the shares in social media are related to female sexual organs
- What do you think about it? Its like drug yeah?
- I started to look at hotels in Thailand etc etc ..island countries are small

CURE

- I can go to make therapy to there
- To the sea and forest..to wilds..
- Politics are empty, let's live our own life
- Will you come with me? :))
- I invite you to minimalism
- You'll be happier if you keep it small
- Now how can I imagine behind the dark black glass cars to space ,to the depths of the soul
- Always busy, always busy with the spirit of imprisoned
- I want to walk
- With my old shoes, under the sun
- And thinking and dreaming..
- Understand and grasp
- And be ready
- What do you think: these aliens came to our world before,when the tech is not developed like that? They came and lived far from human ..Maybe they brought to these animals too here..I see a lot of diffirent residue!
- I'm not working on mentals, I'm working on the brain.
-;)
- https://youtu.be/_ejUYwfWK0U
- Watch very carefully
- The methods mine..if people here will not care about them i will go to others..
- How do I get the patents of them?

- You went ?!

CURE

- :)
- Do not make yourself missed doctor

Rahchan:
- I'm leaving tomorrow morning
- Will be 5 days in europe
- It is good now in Europe
- Nice wines in small bottles
- Have a nice trip
- Eu tr is at peace today
- Rahchan:
- Thanks
- Until evening traning
- But i will escape at 3 pm..
- Enough

Ekrem:
-))
- Run..
- Best of

Rahchan:
- Absolutely
  - You know..

Ekrem:
- Come on, I will install you
- You do not need training
- It's nice to run away
- How nice to walk
- Take a picture and see how it looks
- Share

Ekrem:

- According to the circumstances, the personality traits that the struggle of the individual struggle in this struggle can not be the personality disorder!

- You may be paranoid schizoid or maniac in a different environment if you are normal .. How did you react when you encounter a rhino on the way?

- Does this rhinoceros really belong to this world or does this person belong to this world?

- Is it necessary to distinguish neuroticism from personality disorders?

- I have a thing that can benefit the country by taking a step if we can get the result ...

- You run away? :)

- Rahchan! .. really where and how would you like to live?

- http://m.imdb.com/title/tt1714915/

- Is there a religion you've practiced?

- I do not think so

- I think you should choose a religion and start practicing

- Faith opens up perception

- Sports

- You never mentioned of Spor.

CURE

- Start sports

Rahchan:

- I am doing sports
- Certainly i have religion
- But interesting you are
- I was thinking yesterday to go pilgrimage

Ekrem:

- Muslim?
- Go Hadj
- Sports good for you quit cigaret
- You can read memorize sura?

Rahchan :

- No:I do not know

Ekrem:

- Not good..you need practise

Rahchan:

- Yeah
- I wana read about religions..

Ekrem:

- You need to know what it is.
- What happens when you go to the Hadj?
- Go to Hajj then
- You need to read this book..
- The stories of the Prophets
- Design of hell and paradise
- After death what we will do?
- The story of creation
- Buy Turkish translation and read

CURE

-;)
- Hebrew Tora also i read...
- Look what is the problem in religion for people!
- Habibi
- OK
- Good job

- Now the Gregorian calendar based on the birth of Jesus is born in the year 0 ... what we will the time until the birth of Jesus? ..Remove?.. I will not believe that the new year will enter the year 2019 ... For time settings
- They have set up and manage to time for us..
- We use church calendar
- Time is another ...

- I think these two are lesbian, what do you think?
- https://youtu.be/LcBzVuyk_kM
- Look carefully at the eyes, do you feel the hypnosis for 5 seconds?
- Seriously respond
- I can help you quit cigarette afar from you.
- Tomorrow
- I will sending to set
- If you're ready ...

- Sinful Rahchan
- Sinful Ekrem

- We are sinners
- We must always ask forgiveness
- What about Noah Ship?
- The guilty person is a sinful person. Too hard a be human
- We are always guilty.
- Look at the Adam and Eva
- Apples have committed crime..
- God sent them to world..to crime in the world
- God created a crime machine.
- God test us always...
- Why did not Allah help this Syria?
- Very interesting Europe is like paradise but East like hell..
- I guess God sit and watching us
- I think human came here from another planet to plunder to World
- https://youtu.be/XB-TwbVtA6U
- Final track

- What did Simone find on Sarter?
- I tell you:
- I think Simone is a lesbian.
- Sarter understood and legitimized their relation
- So they look like a couple.
- Sarter was free with women and Simone was free with women
- They can not be revolutionaries

- Libertarian revolution can not be remembered in their name
- These are neurotic
- Their hormones are bad.
- Rotten people
- They can not raise babies
- I'm sorry that we have spent our 68 generations mercilessly with considerations

- Do I confess something?
- Hila will do it again
- Rahchan
- Did you hear that
- Russian great ambassador killed
- It was necessary to eat a lot of bread to get the good news to politics
- Politicians can fuck us for 2 minutes..
- To Simone and Sarter ,and Ayse and Azra pornographers of the their own time :)
- Without newspapers they are big nothing..
- Two toes, three to five lines
- Science
- The devil does not die.
- I declare the aristocratic and the humanitarian types of the slave, who think himself beyond humanity.
- We have no differences.
- The last bomb
- When it comes time

CURE

- I will write it
- What is it?
- htttps://youtu.be/B6zzz_DyrcE
- htttps://youtu.be/wPbTObICN8o
- Watch it..
- We've organized it.
- htttps://youtu.be/ghXOJ9-RGFk
- Last video ..
 - Binaural beats
- Do you have any information for that?
- He yo
- Are you ready!
- I will send you something
- htttps://youtu.be/8gI2_kvEV44
- Achievements
- Free
- By the way i missed you..i will call you soon..
- A new state founded
- Are you aware?
- That blood on the face
- I think it's good.
- Are you still in the Crusade? :))
- As a new alternative alliance will be established.
- The official language will be Russian and Turkish?
- You said that you live to real life ,when i look to your life from here I see falsity in your life .. I am right?
 Rahchan:
-Certainly

Ekrem:

I think it's a lot of..

- Before i allowed to people use me..already now i do not allow them..

- Only my mother and father with me..

- Only they are..

- Who can not use going crazy

- Do you have your brother or something?

- I have mine, but I do not have about 10 years.

- For example, when sis got married..she is dissapeared

- The brother my..Also..

- Even your sisters kids can look to you strange..

- If your brother can not use you ..he can go..

- You are a flower

- Look at the copyright ..i published them in the abroad..

- Paperback

- Ebooks

-;)

- The beginning of the year is today

- My congratulations..

- I decided to go to the Bali in August.

- You'll get rid of me :)

- You must write a story with Ekrem ..

- Come to visit..

Rahchan:

-Bali

-Really?

- You are amazing

Ekrem:

Yes, there is a girl

- I can get married

- She wanna get marry me

- Rahchan, Exactly

- I know her for 2 years

- RASNI

- In August we will meet

- I can open cafe-shop there and fill it with books

- Can i call you?

Rahchan:

-I'm on the new year party

Ekrem:

- What are you doing?

- Crazy!

- Hehe

Rahchan:

-Surprise

-Rituals

Ekrem:

- Look good

- Church rituals

- Is the object of the Turkish custom made by the Byzantine ?

- Turks should stay Shamans ?

CURE

- That Black Grape and Sema always burned the candle in the church ..I remember
- Orpheuses in us!
- The correct application of whatever religion !
- Out side of these applications for me foolish..
- Could you write me some arabic word of your religion?
- :)
- You do not know what it is
- You're not a Muslim.
- That's why i said you that : choose religion
- :)
- Come to the outside be outsider.
- Procrastination kills to productivity

- What was it : In fact, the cult has been a Mesopotamis and has not been seen from west . Anyway, Mesopotamis can be easy , Vinci, Einstein, neurologist and astrologer .. They may go to western for education or even without going there and can be wiz. Because those who steal the their cult with weapons and take it to the west try to sell it to them again..
- So if he steals what belongs to me and tries to sell it to me: his hand turns empty ...
- There is something strange.

Rahchan:

-What are you writing beautiful..

Ekrem:

CURE

- Is it true?

Rahchan:

-You're right

Ekrem:

- I miss you..
- Really i love you
- This girl from Bali..Never leave me alone...
- I love you!
- I feel affinity to you
- Maybe you knew me.
- I miss so much..
- Maybe it's in my head.
- Clean
- What I'm feeling
- This is beautiful.
- To be the one who makes you feel good
- No one told me such a thing.
- The real thing.
- Friendly
- Its my inspiration
- Important
- Its foster to my soul
- If you are filling up to my mind and heart
- Yes
- *
- What's this?
- ?
- Filling someone's mind and heart

- Be in your thoughts
- Look at your image in my mind!
- This is you, you are the in my mind and me in yours
-?
- Magnetic
- It's impossible without feeling...
- G nite
-;)
- Some say it's a quantum
- I can live with you in my head for a lifetime.
- Did you understand?
- How?
- You can cheat to your brain
- Love is fake
- It's a lie.
- I find these girls primitive: why? Because, as a human being,they are too irreverent.They do not answer to messages..They always be in expectation..If they couldnt study that in the school ,think so their family too really primitive
- Sex?
- It's for reproduction.
- If you wanna make baby..work on it for 1-2 months
- Without that Wasted shovel
- Women should use to sex for reproduce ..And live like that..Maybe in the world men are wont be oversexed..Someone programing to them different?

- And we would be a society with a more developed individuals ... the man who thinks always about the leg chest etc can not produce anything

-Women should pay attention to their clothes .. I think in the development areas they should be asexual dressing

- Energy must go to the brain

- https://youtu.be/7p5T156l4tg

- What is mean Rahchan?

- Persian

- What do you think ..your lineage from Persia?

- What you think about real is what you believe in your brain..

- You can do this to another brain

- So Adam ate apple

- Yes, yes, Adam and Eve are ate apples

- I falling love to you..yes..yes..now in my mind there is someone who fall in love

- Placebo effect of words

- At the full moment of real life

- I believe you

- Yes yes yes

- They say..

- They always says: there is a single truth..but they always seperate to ways

- It's not true.And now truths..

- Which is correct?

- Whom do we trust?

- Rahchan..

Rahchan:

-My name is Persian

- Roxanne

Ekrem:

- Glitter

- Light

- Actually, I can remove the race from the shape of your toes

- Are you a glint?

- Dazzling?

- Look at this picture!

- According to this, I am a Roman.

-You ?

- https://youtu.be/UiTfUisKuQM

- Count: I have worked in 25 professions

- I have not only one profession i have 50 professions

- Bad

- In a program that can show the skull bone from the picture, you can take an X-ray shape ... then match it

- Head bone structure shows to race

- I do not know how right

- My race is the from peoples of Kenan

- Saliva DNA constructomus is the most guaranteed

- I mean: my grandma race is, already grandfather Mesopotam ...

CURE

- Now according to the story Adam and Eva came
- They were speaking a single language.
- How did the kids get into each other?
- Now there are hundreds of languages..
- How was the eye pulled out of the black-eyed white yellow variety
- Climate or something.
- But the genetics do not fit us
- Height ,weight, temperament
- Blood red but in all
- The word is -Stranger-very interesting
- Something weird.
- As the languages spoken 1000 years ago disappear
- Egyptian ancestral, hint etc. etc. The languages they speak are perceived as antiquity
- Why can not I understand the current Egyptians?
- Or other antiquity languages
- How did these languages disappear..
- What do you think :they came to here when these technologies that are not very developed, ? ... and then leave?
- And they left something out. And our races discovered something from them and made them technology.
- Imagine that the world has a magnetic field .. for example i call your, even if we have 1000 km between us, you can instantly hear my voice. I can instantly send you an instant message without using any cable!

CURE

- We can not see this magnetic field by eye, we can not hold it by hand, but we can embody it as data on the screen
- We can send and visualize codes
- There are millions of billions of frequencies.
- Billion photon light
- Wireless
- Wireless invisible connection
- Instant communication
- Wireless imaging
- Did we discover these things or how..what do you think? They are our?
- Human now very cosmic?
- This magnetic field is something that belongs to the world.
- Very powerful and usable
- And offers very fast communication
- There's something else.
- This seems to me very primitive
- When I imagine more
- Maybe we can go close
- Hokus pokus sounds like an important sentence to me now
- Wireless is like hocus pocus
- I can say there could be more magical magnetic energy analogs that could be used in the world
- So there is a force for sure.

- If we can find that force.
- Maybe they found it.
- Because instantaneous remote communication can be so fast.
- It's a core thing.
- Could it be people's transportation?
- Reflection of the image can be moved
- Self-contained magnetic field
- Anyway I fly
- Where did I come from to this?
- We do not remember the strange Sumerian preface as the peoples of the world
- Always had strange language and alphabets before or before
- We can remember it as solid as once.
- But there is a disconnect
- Have you ever thought about these?
- What do you think Adam came to World very ignorant?
- Are we the truth ... Are you telling that you are the truth..I m saying that i only seeking to truth..Maybe i m the truth..
- You are my quantum love ...Your image of soul, reflexing to my brains quantum
- Is it in there?
- https://youtu.be/fl65pnNMVzU
- This song will tell you your name very well..

Cansu:

CURE

-Hey ... Ekrem! Wake up .. the season is over ..

-Do you hear me? When I snap my fingers, you can open your eyes.

Ekrem:

- What am I to do? Who are you ?

Cansu:

-I am Cansu! Did you forget me ? ⁇

-Who is the Rahchan?

Ekrem:

- How did you know that?

-What did you do to me, Cansu? I'm lost, I went ..

Cansu:

-You were talking about Rahchan ... ... during the hypnosis ... Who's this Rahchan?

Ekrem:

I do not know, Cansu .. I hear hervoice, I feel her, even someone I can see and can not see. It's someone I can touch, even i can not touch..

Someone who i love,but i cant love , who takes me, but takes me back without letting me stay there, but who takes my mind and who back me my mind..

- Someone filling to my soul with life but discharge it up again and again and filling it up and edischarge it again.. someone who calls me in dreams and takes dreams and hides them in the truth .. I do not know who is this Rahchan .. how I can tell you Cansu ...

- Or is that you, the Rahchan?

Cansu:

-Don't frown -... Come on .. I made you a very delicious coffee .. Come on ..

Ekrem:

-OK..

-Cansu ... I told you about my dreams ... tell me what happens to me?

Cansu:

- You live with one of the Rahchan, Ekrem ...

Ekrem:

-What do we do?

Cansu:

-Do you want to erase this Rahchan from the head? What are you doing with it?What will you do with her?

Ekrem:

- I do not do anything .. She comes and he lives with me ... I can not do anything .. Do I want to be saved? I do not know...

Cansu:

-Come on here and kiss me.

Ekrem:

-What?

Cansu:

-Come here ...

- Your lips are like honey. I want you!

Ekrem:

-Cansu!

Ekrem:

-Ekrem!

Cansu:

- Take me from here Ekrem..

Ekrem:

-Where?

Cansu:

- I do not know..I want to run away and I want to be with you all the time.

Ekrem:

- Let's go, Cansu.

Cansu:

- Let's go..Gods will disappear in the middle of the salt rain of our ages, Somewhere in the blue of the skies that will give my love .. I love you very much Ekrem ..

Ekrem:

-We're going out!

Cansu:

-Are we going ?

Ekrem:

-Yeah, we're going.

Cansu:

- Where we go ?

Ekrem:

-To Idyllic!

Cansu:

-Where is there?

Ekrem:

- Shut up and hold my hands . Follow me silently and watch around.

ANSWER

Artur:

- Something happened....

- The words always tricked and I think you started to think.That's why you did not write anything, so you did cause me to wait.My writing, my words, caused you to make other images on your head and make strange decisions.Nevertheless, I certainly do not mean the images that are formed in your head.I want you to know that.Because we never talked to each other and we were trapped in these white pages.How can we understand each other with the words in these texts ? You read what I write and you always think of other things, thoughts and dreams.Did you draw another me in your head and live him ? Then does my feelings and thoughts go away fly away? Is it disappearing? What kind of transformation is this. We never know each other at all,at the head of everyone there are different like me, like you and like them.. If you love me like that in your thoughts,i m in too..I can be that and you ..in my head ..different you are ..I know that too..I know that my love, who is mine, is passing by you.Close your eyes, I'll see you in the light of the moment.You are so beautiful .Love must be this. You are always on my mind. I get the life energy from you.

- https://youtu.be/ZxbwPiCZRyk

- I'm sending you a pathological track.

- Noone, what happened to with yours Bay ?

- I'm translating that part right now.

- Came to mind

- I am looking for a magazine newspaper where I can write articles.

- Is it something that comes to mind?

- I showed to a translator from a university, she gave 92%

- I am using dictionary too.

- The editorial program gives 74%

CURE

- Teacher gave more than 90%
- I feel better when I do it myself .. everything is perfect, under my control.
- These neo nazis will resurgence again ?
- Anyway, you learned a lot from me, doctor.
- Watch out for left and right.I'm gone for a while.

Noone:
- Artur!
-The Bay is going slow
-They just did not allow Stone
-They do not want construction
-They said that made wood
-I've been trying to produce a different concept
-Glass ,wood and stone
-We will get something out
-Except that one
-I'm knitting
-Very enjoyable
-And meditative
-If i can read some books
-It will be fine
-I can not go to the hospital because of the weather..

Artur:
- You can make a good bay in the direction of opportunities..
- Knitting like meditation for women,now i remember ,i will send you a link ,knitting firm making premiums on knitting designs in England.

- I need to look ..

- Noone,my translation soon will end,well then you will read book,read my translations,i will send you them or read my another book that i send you before..

- I think so ,you do not go to hospital,you can feel better

- :)

- Do not you work from home or something?

- :)

- Wool and the gang

Noone:

-Haaaaa

- I went to their London factory.

Noone:

- I know ...

- Super

Artur:

- Yeah..

- Design it and send them

- They are replicate them and sell..

Noone:

-I did not know that way..

- I have their email address..

Noone:

-But a super concept in the name of wool and knitting..

Artur:

- Yess..

- My ex wife was fashion designer..

CURE

- I took her there.

  Noone:

-Super you are..

Artur:

- They have big shop in the Oxford Street..

  Noone:

-You got every fucking news..

Artur:

- I saw that singer Neriman

- I insulted her.

- It was good anyway.

- There must be Jess.

- https://youtu.be/OjVeMK-spow...

- I opened the stand for that idiot in the full navel of London ... at Portebello and Nothinhill.

- Then I was a schizophrenic, I was gay, what kind of job ;)) ..She talked like that of me..

- No longer ,now she can see that only in her dreams..

- If you were my wife, would you leave me ?

- Be a woman of your house, my daughter :)

- Ha ha

- https://youtu.be/mL4Nhc0b9Yk

- Listen to the bomb of the day

- High quality

- Dj Artur

- Noone!

- English is over 120 pages

- I do not think you want to read today.

- But it was great.
- The end was very beautiful

Noone:

-Very congratulations

-Please send it.

Artur:

- Where do I send it?
- What format do you want?

Noone:

-I will do it

-I like to read on paper

Artur:

- ok..
- A4
- Noone:

-Yes

Artur:

- Email: noone@someone.com?
- I made it 6x9'.
- I will send it like that.
- I will send you a4 ok..

 Noone:

-I do not know how to translate format

-I will print it at the hospital

Artur:

-Ok

- I make an A4 for you
- Is not the email correct?

- Turkish Shakespeare borning from the darkness of the ghetto
- :)) hehe
- I made a4 for you, 123 pages.
- Normally it's 6x9' for the printing press, its 168 pages of books,
- I will send it in a moment
- I sent
- noone@someone.com

Noone:
- Yes
- OK

Ekrem:
- I worked like a donkey for this book
- 32 000 words
- I'm waiting for feedback
- From you
- New adventure:
- After the Sounds from the Unseen...
- Will
- Subliminal Love..
- :)
- You need a good publisher.
- For make some money.
- I have not given a local publisher yet.
- For these books
- Do you have a request from me?

- Today my aunt came and said that : People will be able to travel through the way of light. Look at her what she thinking of.. Actually, I think it's true too.What is wireless, what is electricity, what is magnetic energy ? If they are, there could be a magnetic field that can raise and beam the human body.If we can move our imagery to other areas through electricity, internet and cameras, we can travel at the same speed if we can explore the necessary energy and power fields. There are studies that prove that you can charge a magnetic field and move it to another area..This can bring to mind that the human body can be loaded with maagnetic area and moved to another region at the same speed. I think that it can happen in the electro magnetic environment rather than the irradiation.Something like human mass is loaded and moved to electricity in a magnetic field.You may need a machine for this.Could the human brain be able to do this without being attached to any machine? In other words, with mind power, you can find a new magnetic field and frequency, enter it, move it wherever you want.. As all of your body atoms are broken up quickly and joined another space very quickly. Is this speed of light speed? I think no. It must be a another speed.Yes .. there is that speed .. as if waiting to be discovered.Could it be a visual speed, in which time and space can be found.As a result it can be described as a space because it will be magnetic.It will contain many fractions such as time, speed, etc.The speed we are looking for, when we go to this magnetic field, can be a speed that can meet us in another dimension.I think that our atoms can adapt according to the theory of quantum entanglement.My aunt may be right.

- :)

- I give up from the publisher ,internet enough now

- The recipient can discover ,it will be there forever

- I guess I just need to get the money from the exchange

- Should not be sold with money that is useful to humanity

- Who is seeking can read yeah ?

- I do not want these studies to be commercial.

- I will keep myself back ;)

- Now i remember to one philosophers experience,he said that ,about a philosopher who wrote for the money : Now he is 60 age but he turned into a baby of 4 years..Cos he always wrote for money..

Noone:

-Yes artfully

-Always

-It is

Artur:

-Yeah

Noone:

-Me for last exhibition paid from my pocket

-And I do not sell nor buy it

-I made public

-For the art sake

-And not to participate in all sales-oriented fairs

-I had to this decision
Artur:
- Beautiful
- Right
- For the people
- I think that in the future somebody will find what I write
- So I publish it in a much more postmodern environment, not publisher crocodiles
- And cheapest
- And in 10 - 12 countries
- English for all peoples of the world
- I want you to be lawful.
- Now I see that the singer-guru thinks she's an artist.
- And those who brought her there
- :)
Noone:
-They're trading, honey.
Artur:
-So
- Porno
Noone:
-Trade with Art
-But the broken world
-Now, art is
-In the hands of the idiots..
Artur:
- Unfortunately

- Noone, Art ....

- Pity

- I met with the publishers, no one asked what you wrote, always money always money

- It does not matter what you write.

Noone :

-I always said that how Miro can make a painting for 40 years..

-Miro foundation now sells his copies..

Fuck..

- Strange ..

Artur:

- I sow seedling for future...

- Cos of they are being like monkey when they are old...

- We must call some artists and set up a new art movement..

- Unconsciousness

- Subliminalism

-!

- That famous historian teacher ..There is no other mentor ? What he says ,we must believe? In 2007, we met with my Russian teacher with him for the study of ethnology in the his room Topkapi.I can not tell you how he was a russian speech..He is so abusive..

- I think so his mother is Russian or Ukrainian..

- I do not think there is a real historian in the world..

- I wanna ask you a hardcore question...

- What is the trip of a person having sex in a dream? What is your medical opinion about masturbation?
- Interesting topic
-!
- What can a brain that can do it in the dream do more?
- He's doing unconscious work to the organs ...
- Is this a disorder? Is it that the emptying in the dream is the messenger of a disease?
-!
- At the crack of dawn ..
- It's like you're pissing in a dream when you're a kid.
-?
- Do you have any patients telling you this?
- Could the brain be coded to be able to do this every night?
- Is the control of the organs free when the brain is asleep?
- Is this happening to women?
-!

Noone:

- The brain starts to fall asleep (neither is it a separate topic), the organs assume that the thing on the line is alive and that the reproductive channel starts to work !!! What is it in brain that triggers this broadcast?

Noone:

-In a man who has been in adolescence, the production of sperm (semen water) is continuous and never stops.

These spermatozoa are collected in a sperm pouch and ready to be emptied, and there is continuous sperm production from the back and this sperm pouch is completely emptied, there is a capacity of this sperm pouch, there is a volume, this capacity increases the feeling of fullness in the groin full, and of course, If it does not happen with masturbation, pain in the groin, excessive sexual desire begins.

Even if this process continues but there is no ejaculation, sometimes the purse is so full that the penis sperm flows (this is not ejaculation and does not give pleasure ,only sperm comes) when you poo or the pressure in the body increases.

If the person does not cum or does not make sex, after a certain period of time, the time varies from person to person (average 4 to 10 days), the body is cum when asleep and discharge to sperm pouch to open place the sperm coming from behind.This ejaculation is usually accompanied by erotic dreams. Sometimes these dreams are remembered, and sometimes they are not remembered. In general, a complete relationship can not be established in the dream. It lasts up to old age in men who are active in the sexual orientation and lasts until the loss of sexual power. The frequency of night discharges is proportional to the frequency of discharge (masturbation or sexual intercourse). At the same time, the age varies according to the intensity of the sexual stimuli and the sexual structure (hormone level).

Night dreaming is not a disease, as it is an entirely normal physical emptying.

Artur:

-It's okay.I saw thanks..

- That's for my english book
- I thought I had a few contacts in NY
- Did you get it , Noone?
- Can we create a neuroscience magazine?
- I do not know what those exhibits are,that you paid..?
- If at least we can write something that people can enlighten
- Continuous
- If we start a bow that has scientific, intellectual things ...
- Then we go further ...
- For God's sake, what are you missing from this fancy journalist's lady?
- There's a flare!
- This idiot's making news of rape....There are a lot of important news..
- Why she is always like that..I think that she is really perverted..
- We can make interviews with important people and write of these..
- In the long run we can learn all and we can make you a deputy..You really want to do politics.

Noone:
-Do it..
Artur:
- :)
- Not me ...

- I'm an empty man.
- I know all of them.
- Do you know what i can be ...nothing
- I do not like ties.
- :)
- I do not like navy blue or black suit.

- You are who wants to do something
- Not me..
- If we will create a magazine, I will invest
- I am the writer
- Its not me who is in your head, my lass.
- Change it :)

- Do you think I am sick, or am I trying to open your mind ? ... what do i want from you ? ..Did you really bored from me ? ... or have you always inspired from my thoughts ? ;)
- I'm a philosopher
- I can give you the only ideas
- This is my job...
- I ask you a different question: Let's say your life is very critical and you have problems and you have problems to solve .. I came to you and I told you .. I gave you an idea and you applied it .. You looked at it and it helped to solve the problems This idea saved the burden on you and made you sleep comfortably. What did you give me for this?

- The situation is this: I usually hang out alone.I am reading and writing or going on foot, I am not being with someone ..I can not stand it I can not handle it.. Because with whom I see,i got bad results..I stay away..Because I feel close to you in this respect and I know that your perceptions are strong, you are intelligent and your understanding is good quality..Cos of i do not talk with anyone ..only i talk to you ...From a social perspective its enough for me..Of course its not sicken you.
-!
Noone:
-It does not sicken me
-Unlike.
-You have more knowledge than me in many subjects
-I'm happy to learn..
Artur:
- Ok, I love it.
Noone:
-I lived like a sheep
-I say I know about the world
-There are also some issues
-But there are many issues that I find myself insufficient
-Recent history
-General economic balances
-And global political goals and strategies
-I would like to know
-But there are no people who know these things in my study
-They're all more sheep than me..

Terrible! I felt very bad myself right now ... I lived as empty and lost time. But there was a lot of things I could do. I got up early like an officer in the early hours, went to work and disappeared in my sleep. I had unnecessary fatigues on the ground. I do not think I'm still late. I'm thinking of making new decisions to fix it. You've been very helpful to me to think about it.So glad i have you Artur..

Artur:

- Now my dear Noone: I am a real crazy person who has traveled 35 countries and read an estimated 10 thousand books and I can teach you a lot ...

Noone:

-Social media insights have everyone in snapchat

-They put a dog's ear in their head and leave themselves in a stupid crawl

-Pity all of us.

Artur:

- Have you seen the video of the donkey ?

- I did send you yesterday!

- I said you of we can make a magazine ... or we can write serious writings.

- Let me start politics from there.

Noone:

-Teach me what you know. I read with great interest

-These are the topics that I mentioned before.

-It's about wanting to know my world

-Everyone is looking for a jape..

-This is the collapse of human capital. I'm ashamed of my humanity. I really want to do something serious. Sometimes I think that I am a self-sabot or something. But what I think it might be useful to think about and try to do is why it is a sabotage then I say. I am aware of this change that I am now. Being confronted with new information turned into a kind of social phobia episode. It seems to me ... I get used to it. Perhaps it is a new awakening for me and I have to drink a coffee to come to myself.

Artur:

- Go drink your coffee Noone

- With political scientists and strategists..

- Things I know:

- I have mastered politics, I can teach

- Diplomacy teaching

- Finance

- Military strategy

Noone:

-Current rising trend is addiction

-System fool us

-Its their new move

-Just like the Indians

-Like they're fooling around with alcohol

Artur:

- What did they do to the red-skinned you know ?

- When the Indians saw the bearded people from the sea

- They thought that they are the God..
- Did you know that?

Noone:

-Nooo..

- It is..
- When they saw the first bearded man ,they said that our gods came from the sea..
- They gave everything.
- Look at the perception.

Noone:

-There are no differences from us..Look at to our wannabe ! Look how the culture is formed in loop.We want to take our share as if something has happened from this transformation.But we are not even aware of the anguish that lies beneath what looks like this magnificent.Life philosophies that arise as a result of hardships,Should I not understand that? It seems to me that we have to adapt to something.In some way, it is necessary to have a secular authority.There is a fundamental authority, no matter how numerous it seems..We can not get out of it.This will continues always..Only the old decor is changing ..As time progresses, we continue to share the same anguish in the more advanced decor.We are still hungry again, we want to sleep again, fall in love, share and prove ourselves.

Artur:

- Women with red skin stretched by the cross came to mind now.
- American history

Noone:

-Some of us sell to us fake modern democracy.

-Or an idea ...

-On the other hand, we give everything we have. We are very cruel. In fact, while we see ourselves very democratic, some of us sleep and someone take to a large part of the pastry. We just return from work in the evening, lean back to our canapes,Unaware of anything and we can only watch on TV .It is a philosophy of life, a philosophy of life that designed by others and a philosophy of life we have to obey. Designed outside of the laws of nature.They have been prepared and put into practice without asking us.It seems to be losing my belief in some things when I think of a person or people who preparing them.But nothing to do.It is because they have driven us with survival instinct. We have to fight with it.How did the first man start his first day in the world and with which life philosophy and law? Could it have been possible? I guess he got adapt.Cos he did provide proliferate..These thoughts always inspire me to think of death and after death.Millions of meaningless questions and thoughts are wandering in my mind. Even though I get up early in the morning and go to work, I go home and finish all the routine work I have to do.I am aware that time is progressing and I am getting old.My children are aging in front of my eyes.Interception, fear and pride surround me all while I watch them.It is really this war of survival.Others, however, always pursue an order, battling war, breaking down the old style and building new ones.I know that i am ineffective here.I also know that i will never have an effect on these things.There is a pressure on me that I should be satisfied with what is given to me.This is what I should be doing.Because I usually feel the same things I do in the day, and everyone feels something like what I feel.I also watch people , they are dying one by one. I have never seen anyone come back. It sounds like a metaphysical loop. People are born, living and dying, it's like real order. Other than that, things like management schemes designed, life philosophies, religious ideas, arts, thought, self-assurance, achievements, sons, mothers, fathers, political tendencies and everything just change and develop in life. It is as if the world and nature have a much harder law outside us than we designed.From this point of view, I think that we need to study this situation better and understand it.I understand that the meaning of nature is much more than the meaning of life.We try to understand the facts in life and death cycle and we can really get ready for later.Maybe it's what everyone wants to understand, but nobody even wants to think about it because it's easier to escape. Maybe all the fun, to get close to this mystery. I started to think and lift my head to the sky.My thoughts might come to you very pessimistically Artur..But maybe it might be close to the truth.It's like a human crying at birth.For the surroundings great pleasure the baby to be born,but the baby is coming to the world crying. We can perceive the pessimistic thought positively, not negative. It can help us see the right things. Of course, it depends on what we want to see and not see.

Artur:

- Dear Noone, I recommend you and will tell you three books that you should read and finish.Ok? Later on: I think that you can increase the capacity even more in such things as fast comprehension of information, fast reading etc. and more analytical thinking ..

- What do you think ?

- Take these books and start reading now:

-1.Artur Shopenhauer-Parerga and Paralipomena

-2.Artur Shopenhauer-The World as Will and Representation

-3.Artur Shopenhauer-Aphorisms

- When you finish them ..Let's talk about it;

Noone:

-Okey

- Do this..

- A wonderful start for you

-If you look at it, it will be the capacity to read 20 books in 2 months

- These books that will quickly bring you back 7 to 8 years I think you have spent

- When was the last time you read a poem?

-The poetry is the top spot of art..

- A wonderful start for you

-If you look at it, it will be the capacity to read 20 books in 2 months

- These books that will quickly bring you back 7 to 8 years I think you have spent
- When was the last time you read a poem?
- The crown is the top spot of art
- It looks like
- Your voice is beautiful and you should sing sometimes
- Did anyone ever say that your voice is beautiful?
- I think it's very effective.
- Do you know what I did to the stupid reporter? In instagram?
- In the morning, with a butcher in the middle of the meat, she was making a advertising of the butcher. The shredded meats are flying around, she was near the butcher.
- :)
- 1 day ago she was sharing her house in India, there were sculptures of cow paintings all over the house and so on. It was her respect to Buddha..
- I said the woman your Indian friends should see your photo of you with the butcher .
- Then she started to share her pictures with Indian people..
- I wrote it down so you can have a barbecue with them..
- She answered me that : - do not look a gift horse in the mouth .It is a womanly reaction, as a man has perceived another. She did not understand that I mean some religious ritual.
- :)

- If Indian people can see these photos ,they can bury her in the navel of India

-;)

- Bitch

- I want to capture the media

- :)

- They should stay hungry,then can go to the house in India, they can advertise chop.

- Do you know why you worshiped this cow ?

- This woman is live very good , the poor people are just looking ..

- Oh how nice ...

- Yesterday you said, make animations of a cat and a dog, give to people them on internet ..just enough for the nation.

- Society!

- What was ? 100 people was sucking the blood of a state.

- They were showing us photos in the magazines.

- They were noble

- Elite..

- Because it's money.

- What difference do we have

- How vampire is it?

- They humiliated everyone.

- If you sitting with them ,they can not give you two or three words, then they deserves to direct me about any subject.

CURE

- I'm afraid it's over.
-;)
- We live the caste system.? You discriminate us ?
- Look at the filthy.. nations have lived this for years.
- I find the upcountry more elite, at least they knows the essence.
- I deserve Darwin sometimes.
- :)
- Some like monkeys.
- I'm aggressive now;)
- Relatives, what do you think about ...
- Why they do not like each other
- Because they have common heritage?
- I look at my aunts and with my mommy and they are always in a race..

- Why would the family want to be the most popular ...
- They come together just for a day and then they do not talk for long.
- And always a pragmatism...envy..
- What is motherinlaw ? Mother does not love bride and can not share her son..
- She always Intervenes..
- Very high gossip..
- Relatives do not like each other and are jealous.
- And they do not help..
- And they say that : we are devout people..
- They know how to disgrace.

CURE

- Because of this, when you marry a woman, you are married to her family too..
- Hard work
- I can not
-;)
- How difficult are they doing?
- You take the Russian chick, you sit in the middle of the room, you take care of the sun, and you see uncle's, dad starting to cut this chick!
- If they can catch her alone ,they can fuck her..do not care Artur their :)
- Haha..I think world is bitch..
- 95% of the relationships are pragmatic.
- Trying to put feelings into mind and exploiting
- It depends on mind games.
- Dear Noone .
- The number of intelligent women is very low
- Or you do not know what's in you.
- Why should I envy a woman? Look at obsesion.
- How is my translation?
- Actually, the book seems to be written in English again.
- 60,000 words
- Jealousy is the show of love ?
- it's a sign of a obsession ?
- The women steal one's heart in the bed.
-!
- Hunter women.

- So if you make a compromise on yourself to make me jealous, it's not worth any more in front of my eyes.
- Meaningless attempts
- Nobody expects any proof.
- I do not need to try to make something that will end up in bed so valuable :)
- Ohh so beautiful, I love you my love.. give me suffer ..
- Look at sadism..
- You must stop talking to her again, this is fucking crazy.
- I am writing "Who is talking", but the Broken Mirror's translation will take 10 days
- Then I will go to for 1 - 2 months and look at the south in a place, a place where I can live and work.
- I do not want to take these colds in the winter
- Lofty thing ,I gotta do is the cheapest part of the sea
- I will write 10 -15 books
- Can be Izmir
- It makes sense.
- Cheap and calm
- Do you know Izmir well?
- I was a soldier there.
- Like this entrance, there are places like the loft shop?
- Talk to me !

- Whats up ?
- I have written a heavy book. The Turkish language is over 230 pages of English which is 195 pages.
- It's a very good book.

CURE

- A fairly philosophical
- Writing does not make money, it's super.
- What was the first thing people ate when the world first came?
- Was it the poor ,the first person?
- Was the first person to come naked in the world?
- Dear Noone: sometimes I know you can not fully perceive what I write.
- I met a girl, Slovak.
- Smart
- But he wants to dominate a man :)
- This stupid side
- But I do not take that role.
- She is beautiful.
- Archaeologist.
- She bumps the wall.
- I remember: Master for Hegel said that he was writing for the money.
- Do i need to look at the sky to understand the world? I had a telescope sometime. I gave that to my nephew 7 ~ 8 year old .Now he should have strange world.When he see me ,he admire me..Think ,Eye of a seven-year-old child looking out over a pipe with optic lenses at the tip.He sees the stars and planets hidden in the darkness.God knows how thrilled his heart.This excitement will stay in his subconscious.I hope he will be able to do more in the future.I wanted him to be his a beautiful dreamland.Sometimes I can see he imitate me.That's a good thing.Maybe there will be a lot of

things he can talk to me in the future.Maybe he will always remember me when he looks at the stars in the dark.

-Noone, you made this mood disorder a gum on my dad's mouth.Fix it..

- If this goes on like that, I'll start to swear at your back.

- You called him for your own trouble, you bothered me with the way it worked out. fix it ...clean ... You just diagnosed to me from 600 km away.I am angry to you..

Noone:

-Yes, you get angry to me

- I can fix it..

- What about talking your father?

Artur:

- He says that i have bipolar..

- And i am sick and i do not accept this..

- I'm nervous that you put this on me, I have to defend the accusations that are not correct when I have a breakfast..

- And this is the workplace..

- I say him that I am a writer.

- He tells me about the writer's head to be a writer, and i think so the editors are the most idiots of this world.

- Something or something.

- Under his subconscious want to see evidence that I'm doing something and being like he wants .

- He has the real anxiety..

- I ask him that please tell me of Epic Gılgamesh ..

- He escaped..

CURE

- That time do not say me that you can not writer..

- His experiences taken in the training of this old classical civil servant motivation program 1980 model ..

- I can not work somewhere, do not get married again, just live and live for life. I will soon go from home again..

- I like İzmir I want a warm place like İzmir in 1-2 years. I can not do it in the same place with people for a long time .. They are releasing very empty and unnecessary negativ..

- He was cancer, he always thinking of death

- You actually give him a biotherapy

- A medication

- You can tell him that everyone already dying

- If you realize that 250 years of tearing your butt will not have the same life head in this world

- I know that I am not in a place where I would be delighted to be a person with the concept of death and meaningless in my 20s

- I can take a drug every day..

- Ha ha ...

- Anyway, take him away from me. Turn him back to the previous factory settings. Tell him what it is on me do not understand or anything. Tell him about me that i am the alien or something.

- Tell him that me must keep writing.

- He is asking me what you are writing ,i say of neuro science and metaphysics

- And then he talks about his successes
- I always say politicians are empty-headed, including my father
- I have to go in a little while.
- It's close.
- Although he always keeps to mom back, the woman is smarter and her world is more fantastic ..
- Their brain was hackled in 68.
- There's nothing left to give to the next generation.
- If they were intelligent, they would continue their training in the libraries as they would not attack each other in university corridors
- This is the life style intervention
- What the family did to the child
- Let the child choose
- You do not do this to your children.
-If you want to bring a child to the world, you must do what kids want?
-The kid does not have to do anything at all
- Kid came for what you wanted
- If they asked me that would you like to come to world..i would say no..
- There's a high-level mobbing at workplaces
- Noone can not come together..
-Do you think we can distribute high-level understanding?

Nooone:

- In our country there is to high formalism..With this formalism,Trying to get into these people, try to hold on to life, like try to walk without using an oxygen cylinder on the moon.There is always misunderstood, it is defined as what you are not, and trying to defend that it is not what you are not. Hugging to white lies does not relieve me too much.People are afraid to open their mouth.Maybe that's why I hug the cigarette.Too much chaotic everything, you turn on the TV, constantly violent news, suffering people, weapons, explosions, and you are going to work,to there unlimited desires, people who work with limited resources, fake success motivations.Love comes to your mind and, unlimited expectation shoot to your brain.What is this test, trial, trust, insecurity? Am I a trial board? It is really fag out. When everyone wants to have what they want, how can we compromise ? I think that social psychology is a collapse.The fact that there is a continuous system update indicates that the existing system is still inadequate.I mean either unlimited desires and limited resource..we need to people who can make a limit to unlimited tenderness and adapt to limited resources.If we accept everything as it should be and not as we want it to be,Would it be bad? People do not push each other's capacities. In this point, mental science is also insufficient.The mood of a person constantly changes, mutation is going on.Every change is a behavioral disorder, followed by a new anti-depressant.

So while the mood is constantly in an unlimited desire. While the body is mutating, the soul and the brain are also mutating. Because of this, the system keeps updating itself constantly. I am very curious what kind of entity will be in the future.I see that this development took place in the last 50 years. If this development continues at the same pace in the next 50 years, a much more interesting human race will appear.This change brings with it a lot of diseases.Cancer, HIV and many other diseases are still untreatable.But after this treatment process gets positive results, a certain development process of human beings will come to an end.So a new process will begin.Even today's technology, which we are using now and which we think is of high quality, will lose its value and will be known as primitive technology.If the computers and phones that we used up to 10 years ago are primitive now, after 10 years current tech will be able to take place in our memory..Every change comes with universal illnesses, and when the change is over, it will end and it will be replaced.I think drugs will not come out of our lives if chemistry exists.

Artur:

- An American and New Zealander

- That have read my book.

- One of American is Zoo scientist..

- He has a photograph with a rhinoceros. He also taken my poetry book

- Look

- I made an analysis of behavior in the book after encountering a rhino.He send me an email of that..

- My book Lost Philosopher too will be hardcore..

- I said before,, including my father,noone not take no account of to my books in this country..I will blow outside..

Noone:

-Exit out

-Why not be inside

-But you are in front of time

Artur:

- Nobody reads books here..

- And everyone is looking at the money

- He's taken ...

- He added me in the instagram

Noone:

- Super

- He also took the poetry book

- It's more important.

- Nobody read poetry here..

- I translated everything into English ...

- Lost Philosopher now: this philosophy book is mine..hard..loop is slow..i could translate 6000 words..60 000 will.

- I have difficulties in religion.

- They can attack

-!

- Take your son a telescope! Is there?

- https://youtu.be/nkc84kUthfo

- Dear Noone: Let's say I am FED , for the first time I have strike 1 million dollars. I gave it to the debt-seeking states with 10% interest. They should give me 1.1 million back. But I did 1 million prints. How will they find + 100 000 dollars?

- Again they wanted to borrow 1 000 000 more 10% interest rate
- Total debts were 2 200 000. But what is going to happen here is 2 000 000 returning on the market .. + 200 000 what happens? There's always a debt.
- The world always has debt to the FED..
- They should give gold and sources
- It does not walk without a dollar.
- If there are those who oppose it, they should all strike a new money and circulate it .
- Like the euro.
- East does it ...
- Does not work for anyone
- Prophets have made a great revolution in the economy, in fact they have revolutionary sides by forbidding interest.
- How to provide a dollar reserve, whether you will use the resources to produce and export or the central bank will get the debt dendened..Dollar can not step out..You want to learn finance .. I said a bit.
- https://youtu.be/O2Gs2EXm-MM
- Can you listen to the songs I sent you, doctor?
- You know the intensity of what I'm writing ...
- Are you postponing books?
- Now i see , why are the peasants pure..

- Hey Noone: what would be the worst thing you could do to get revenge on a man as a woman?
- I think you were leaving him.
- Much more?
- When you leave, are you taking revenge?
- That Reina killer
- A good I catch.
- Look at the police who worked so well.
- Because he cheated on his wife.The wife has sell him away.Look at the revenge..
- I send you one smile today :)
- I can not send a heart.Sorry i need it..
- There's a real steak tartar a la turca
- Do you want to?
- :)
-Noone, what do you think of lechers ?
- These types
- What medal do we give them ?
- https://youtu.be/0CWVgu2Odjg
- You heard gold production increased.
- Demand increased
- We're doing analysis 2 days ago

Noone:
-I need to find gold mine.

Artur:
- Yeah
- But look, there's still interest.
- Strange things come to mind..

CURE

-There are not usually paper money in anybody's pocket .. big money .. everyone keeps the money in the bank ..

- There are only cards in their wallets

- And they sees his money on digital screens.

- The cash money in the somewhere in the warehouses..

- You do not know if the banks have moved it to another place

- you're stuck with your credit card

- You can pull up to 5000 by ATMs.

- Everything is digital

- Now if people say we will take all of our money from the banks

- Can all of this money be taken out of all the banks?

- It's just stay interest debtors then?

- Interest

- The banks can only attack them.

- But it can all over for the banks

.- It seems like the money is moving out of the country or the stock market, etc.

- So it keeps shaking up the exchange rate

- There is something that is not replaced.

- In this storage

- In my opinion..

- It's a borrowing I think, a secret dollar borrowing

- We do not know how to move money.

-!

- How is this money in a crazy atmosphere?

- The guys have made space.

- Look at the system ...
- Where is the gold that is said to exist in the same way?
- Hiding or standing somewhere!
- Hey Noone: what do you call women born with a male organ? What kind of formation is this?   She comes out like a woman, but she has a masculinity organ.
- They say to them shemale.
- It's interesting
- They are hiding themselves most of the time, but recently they have begun to appear a little bit
- No religion does not explain their situation.
- These are the third kind? What are you saying..?
- I wonder about this comment
- A scientific look, please.
- How do I come to you?
- This is kind of ... how would it be if she was a child? Noone:

-Yes, things like that, yeah Artur..Hermaphrodite, Test feminization .. and other endocrine diseases .. Developmental disorders in the genital organs are caused by genetic disorders, hormonal disorders (fetal endocrine disorders), or emriological disorders occurring during development of the genital organs.In order to be able to understand sexual and sexual development anomalies more easily, it is necessary to pay close attention to normal sexual differentiation Artur. First, the undifferentiated gonads appear as the first outline of the embryonic period in front of the Coelomic epithelium 4-5 weeks. Within this draft, the cortex and medulla later appear.When the medulla develop in the male, the cortex becomes a represse.In the female kortex develop and medulla becomes a represse.The yolk sac follicle is one of the important steps in the gonadal embryonic development of primordial ferm cells (5-6 weeks).If this does not happen, the gonads can not complete the development, the gonadal agenesis develops and the ovaries remain in a band (streak gonad). It is the genetic characteristic of the person who determines the gonadal differentiation mainly in male or female.Only the XX chromosome is sufficient for the development of ovaries.If the gonad is not already alerted, it is programmed to differentiate in the female direction.A special warning is needed for gonadal differentiation in a male fetus. This warning is TDF with HY antigen in Y chromosome.The internal genital system is known to occur in the channels of Wolf and Müller.Differentiation in the male direction, medullary gonads develop in the presence of Y chromosome and differentiation in the testis direction.The testosterone hormone released from the testis allows the wolf channel to differentiate in the direction of the epididymous vesicles semidis and vas conferences. In addition, MIF (Mullorian duct inhibiting substance) released from the testis causes suppression of the müller duct. In the absence of MIF, Müller develops into the canal and will form Tubas, Uterus and Vagine 2/3 above.In the absence of functional testes the internal genital system will develop in the female direction.Outer genital organs with development potency on both male and female sides include urogenital sinus, labioscrotal folds, and genital tubercles.As the inner genital organs are in development, if the stimulus does not come here, the female develops.The labium, clitoris and 1/3 lower part of the vagina occur.For male, the warning is the testosterone itself.However, in order to differentiate the external genital organs, testosterone must be converted to DHT (dehydrotestosterone) via the 5 ∞ reductase enzyme in the peripheral tissue.It is the DHT that allows the external genitalia to differentiate in the male. With this hormone effect, the genital tubercle becomes to penis, labioscrotal folds scrotum and urogenital sinus urethra and prostate.If there is not enough testosterone production, or if there is a defect in the 5 ∞ reductase enzyme system, then there is no androgenic stimulation and the female develops.Thus, the genital tubercle become to clitoris labioscrotal folds become to labium majusa and urogenital sinus to labium minis.If the female fetus is exposed to adverse events during the critical development period, there may be maskulogenation (masculinity) at different levels in the external genitalia.(Clitoral hypertrophy, labium scrotalike resemblance).The gonads of these cases do not contain MIF if they have female characteristics and the müller develops in the channel, the internal genital organs are female. If there is not enough androgenic activity in the male embryo until the 12th week, the development of the male genitalia can not be enough.

46 XX and female do not develop as normal females, although they have differentiated gonads. Ethiologic genetic, teratogenic factors and gene mutations play a role.When 21 cystoxylase, 11-β hydroxylase and 3 β-

dehydrogenase deficiencies that play a role in the biosynthesis of adrenal hormones are inadequate to produce adrenal cortisol, the pituitary ACTH release is increased. With the increase of ACTH, the precursors of cortisol are increased, and then androgen production takes place. As a result, the effort to raise the cortisol level of the organism results in high amounts of androgen production.

- And, Artur, there is male pseudohermophroditism,

There are genetic (XY) testes, but external genital organs do not develop normal male type, they are mostly female. Gonads are testes and produce testosterone. In these patients, there is no androgenic flesh and the feminine sign develops in the target tissues due to the absence of androgen receptors or the enzyme that converts testosterone into dehydrotestosterone. Puberty is not seen in these patients. The uterus is absent and the vagina is not a well-developed .The breast develops as in normal women because testosterone turns into peripheral fatty tissue and estradiol as anomalies in the breast. Gonads or testes are in abdominal or inguinal canal. All hormonal values are in normal male findings. Karyotype should be done to give certainty to the diagnosis. In these patients carrying Y chromosome 20% gonad malgnite (dysgerminoma), gonads ovaries should be removed when there is a risk of cancer transformation. However, the risk of conversion to cancer is apparent after 20 years of age. Once the ovaries are removed, hormone replacement therapy should be performed in these patients and vagina (neovagene) should be surgically performed in sexual function.Some patients have partial androgen insensitivity.These are the types of puberty women.These are the types of puberty women, but clitoris growth can be seen as hypospadias labuschrotal fusion. In these cases, syndromes such as dums, gibert-Droyfus and Reiffnstein have been defined.

- I have a little word on you of Turner Syndrome,

In some cases of Turner's syndrome there are no X chromosomal bodies, so names like "gonodal disgenezis", "gonodal agenesis", "gonodal aplazia" are given.The partial or complete loss of the X chromosome leads to this syndrome. Most cases of Turner syndrome are lost in intrauterine life when they are in their mother's womb.In zygotes, the incidence of these chromosomal anomalies is 0.8%, and 3% of them have live births. It is estimated that the incidence of this disease is 1/5000.Gonads are called "streak" gonads because they are seen as fibrous structures in this syndrome and have primer amenore.Temporal shortening is characterized by transient congenital lymph edema in the hands and feet, hypoplasic nipples, chest , distinctive ears, narrow maxilla and palate, small mandibula, epicortus, short and mane neck, kubitis valgus, medial tibial exostosis, metatarsal and metakorplas.Shortness can be seen on the fourth and fifth fingers. Renal anomalies and aorta coagulation, hearing impairment, diabetes mellitus, hashimoto thyroiditis and color blindness are more common than the normal population.

Intelligence development is nevertheless normal, but perceptions and motor organization problems can be seen in patients.FSH, LH levels are above 30 miu / ml and estradiol values are below 20 miu / ml. Make a definitive diagnosis with chromosome analysis.Hormone treatment is given, but since this treatment leads to the fusion of the epiphyses, it is more appropriate to start after the treatment height has stopped, or to keep the estrogen dose low first.

-Artur in the end I will try to explain to you what is real Hermaphroditism:

Hermaphroditism (dual gender) is a combination of female and male phenotypic (external appearance) features. If the tissues of the testis and ovary coexist, it is called true hemofrodism. In the majority of patients, chorioiotomy is 46 XX.Etiology in hermaphrodism is uncertain, but it is common for some of the patients to have mosaicism (the formation of a living thing's tissues by combining two different zygotes).In these patients it is thought that the translocation of a part of a Y chromosome in one of the X chromosomes is defective in the etiology.For the diagnosis of true hermaphroditism, it is necessary to show in the over to follicles and well differentiated testis tissue.Rarely on one side is the testis and on the other side is over.There is 90% abnormal uterus, usually breast development is normal. There is Ambigius genitalia (both male and female genitalia present together). In cases of true hermaphrodism, the aim of treatment is to gain the most appropriate features for external appearance and the patient's upbringing. For this purpose, operations and hormone treatments can be used. Since gonads have a high risk of developing neoplasia (cancer) in the future, they should be removed after sexual development is completed. I hope it is illuminated Artur ..

Artur:

- It's the disease.

- But all healthy

- Have you ever been to these kind of patients?

- Is it really disease or is there a genetic structure like this?

- They are always be reproduced

- When was awared this the first time in the world?

- 3th type human..

- When i open this topic people escape from me :)

- I asked to my mom and she gave a strange answer: - God's miracle is ,creating so, what did you think?

- Shemale is natural when she is with a normal woman

- But is it like being abnormal with a guy?

- What kind of thing Embrio

- Nature law

- There may have been some geneticists made some in the past

- Atlantis, for example.

- Could they have done something inherited?

- There is also a myth in old kabala says of reproduction human and non-human.

- It's not exactly Kabbalah.

- There are these kinds of things described in the passage until the flood of Noah
- Strange
- Can artificial enzymes be produced?
- How can we determine optimal body temperature for enzymes and keep this heat data at the same level? Is there a way to do it yourself?
- Babies born to girls in the Dominican Republic are turning into a man after 12 years old.
- After 12 years, the enzyme needed to turn into a man starts to be secreted.
- They are born with XY chromosome
- Everything starts right on your belly ..
- Thank you for sharing this information with me. Thanks for sharing your knowledge with me.
-Always Artur ..
- Should I handcuff me to their own literature chairs?
- It will not inflate me again.
- Hey Noone: an aforism to you:
"I think that political considerations of all political parties have become dogmatic. Everyone worshipes their party as a religion."
- I think idealism is a rotten apple, its tinpot. Idealist brain = writhing brain..
- Pharaoh in Egypt had become ruler, then he thought he was a god
- It seems as if it applies to all political leaders
- Look at to President
- He walks like God

- The former president seems to be crying because of it!
- Wells always follow the system, the bad ones oppose to the system. It starts with the devil.
- I'm getting extrinsic cosmic signals from these stories.
- What do you think of Cosmos?
- Photons and magnetic waves.
- Signals
- Why did God want other creatures to prostrate human?
- It's kind of Allegiance..
- :)
- I wish we were in conversation with them.
- It's as if people think of themselves as gods ...Now i can see this very nice..
- Could it be that we can rule the other realms ?
- https://youtu.be/mxohhIg5CvE

- Hey Noone: as a reader reading my books, for which feature did you suggest me to others?
- I have decided to remove the Turkish language of books, they will all be English.
- Do not think you are a god in these famous people too!
- When somebody does not recognize them in an environment, they can go to the toilet and look in the mirror and cry.
- That's the rating!
- I tried it on a famous model! ..
- Bond requests have increased

CURE

- Foreign investment
- US and UK
- !!!
- Strange affairs
- This order does not change.

Noone:
-Describe the last sentence Artur ..

Artur:
- Treasury bonds
- State makes new debt securities

Noone:
- ???

Artur:
- Foreign businessmen have bought their estates
- Treasury sells government bonds
- It's a job guarantee.
- Work can be done in this country
- Trust in the state.
- This bond that will pay interest extra ...
- They will also invest

Noone:
-Artur!
 - You understand everything.

Artur:
- I am reading a lot ... and I am a graduate of economics.
- A little bit of economics and statistics by myself
-!

- So you would say that when you propose me that :he understands every other shit ...

This is the profession: The philosopher.

-!

- Prof.Dr.Artur :)))

- Ha ha ...

- Hey Noone: what should we do with my sub-method?

- In developed countries, physicists, quantum and so on. When they are clogged, they apply to philosophers!

- Then we worked, too.

- If I can change your point of view, doctor, happy to me!

- Sub-method, using subliminal and binaural sound systems, after hypnotizing the patient,During the hypnosis, the brain activates the self-scanning function to find the problem.But this is not limited to these binaural and subliminal sounds,There is also brain activation with extra biomagnetic energy using the brain power and with hands.After the brain has scanned itself and found the problem, it has the power to solve the problem itself.I have had a chance to test for asthmatic children, but I have not had a chance to practice because of some rules of your clinic. I will teach you for some days .. Try it in patients.I got a positive result for my work on panic attack.

- The question is whether media can create a dogmatic perspective with perception management! Some channels, for instance, seem to be well aware of this

- If we can see what we are stuck in, we can go out at once, as if we are in the way of seeing the true.

-!

- Harsh realm ..

- You have to read history
- You know politics when you know history.
- Because history repeats itself all the time.
- Easy job..
- The history does not satisfy me very much.
- But I've read quite a bit ...
- Bureaucratic oligarchy
- Look at to this word..
- It means that you need a lot of money to be a politician.
- Because people can use themselves very well for money.
- If you have a lot of money, they can even start to worship you
-!
- This is the system
- Make a lot of money, if you wanna be politics..
- Look this rich man, in the one night, for him all imbecils in the streets.
- https://youtu.be/E-yz11HQtg8
- You must feed people
- Hard to direct the guy without paying the price
- Dirty jobs..
- Every people cry for money..

- But when you go to their side with a blonde Russian woman,You can stay in amazement.

- Ha ha ...

- Son of a bitch.

- What do you think ... what happened to those love hurts in these environments?

- Noone?

- It sounds boring to people.

- What makes people forget ... what is not forgotten ..

- A channel is made about a documentary orangotan

- The behavior of those oranges is very similar to those who have that documentary!

- They're still trying to make the theory of evolution live.

- Look at the management of isolated perception in the field.

- Hey Noone: what do you think about sitting and planning a sophisticated management system, a system of thinking and write a book for the future?

- You shut up the conversation again.

- Hey !

- Hey make a comment for this please : - It finds the exit points in a lot of real dream situations where the power of logic is not enough to suppress the power, the place where the concepts of metaphysical phenomena find their meanings in the intellectual world of the It is also a dream world.The dreams revive in this world, you can connect to God from here! A lot of concepts that are not smart minds are found in the world of imagination.I think it is wrong to think that the broken dreams have such a heavy shocks in the world of imagination that a lot of things that people can not understand.Here Logic is too poor.In this context, the significance of many concepts that are understood in the imagination according to the meanings of the physical environment will also come to the agenda.I think that the only real conceivable concepts are hidden in the Imaginary world, and the facts in the outside world are just as the same dreams.

- Can you call me when you are available?

- I want to ask something..

- It's very useful for people to think I'm crazy

- More freedom

- Best camouflage for the current environment

- When I talked to you, I realized that this placebo effect is used in social media and perception management is done ..

- It's done!

- You will keep the people you know and insulate yourself as much as you can on social media

- Noone ,you are very tired ,think so ..

- I have a remote touch

- How many days can you get a permit or something?

- I think you should live like a woman.

- Feminine, like a mother..

- This is natural.

- What do you think is the top of your work physique?

- What are you saying ;)

- I look at housewives and the are mentally more fit and happiness
- They're having fun..
- Be a peasant, really.
- Super elite
- https://youtu.be/AY002EbA9DI
- This song ..you will like
- You are the second Mor
- Ha ha
- Freud said before that he could not solve the soul but i will show him all the world in my next book ..
- You are a old frump ..
- Ha ha ...
- https://www.amazon.co.uk/dp/1520425724
- Take this
- Just mine..
- Published
- Become a member to amazon
- Then take a photo with it and send it to me.
- You can suggest to your friends too..
- I want you to read.
- Cover design is mine.
- Take this book ... what you can do for me ... then I will try to teach you some meanings that you have not really noticed in the future
- A final analysis: the duration of conversation on the phone is limited, so you have to go from one topic to another quickly. If you have already missed one topic,

the subject that is in the past has already lost its validity for me. . This type of people should listen well for correct diagnosis;

- Your job is too hard ..

- You've gotten used to a complicated, ongoing work.Is it also affecting the relationship with people in this social life? I can not take a big time for a stranger ... but I can not take a long time for something .. I think this is the reason for the procrastination..

- Procrastination!

- Programmed brain ..

- Look at the dependency

Noone:

- Oha

-!

Artur:

- Professional deformation ...

- https://youtu.be/1NafxmI7HAM

- Когда это читаешь как чувствуешь себя?

- Уже по русски буду писать тебе..практику сделаю..закончил все книг писать на англиском и публиковал..а сейчас начинаться буду их переводить на русском.

- Долгое дело но все равно получиться :)

- Пойдет не плохо..

- When you look this Russian text ,very strange yea not understanding?

- Look at the barrage of people!

- That's what you feel when you look at this Russian article, it is me..

- Hey, Noone, look at the type of fish animal.

- https://youtu.be/V3xczgi9Hms

- Look at your key.

- New projects now

- That fish animal refute evolution with his presence

- I have an American plan.

- Noone,

- I can see if the vision is over again.

- A little warm weather

- I want to do NY

- In a Jewish neighborhood

- New Yorker was published on 3-4 poems. 6 photo artworks were bought in Vermont ... I have a friend, there is a gallery there .. He was brought me money from USA ..We went to autistic children together..and i gave this money to them ..He just looked at me very long..

- Lost Philosopher

- Exactly me

Look at the energy of life coming from the combination of 2 hydrogen atoms and 1 oxygen atom

- What color is water color

- Transparency

- And water's living things

- We can discover Creation from the inside

- You can not miss a metaphysical, spiritual point here

These two atoms can not come together randomly while standing
-The color that emerges
- Taste too
- The most delicious beverage in the world
- All chemical experiments with water
- Water's everywhere.
- Mother's womb in fetal water
- It's the same as there is a difference in salt water in the sea.
- I'm entering chemistry soon
- I will send you a biography clip
- https://youtu.be/5_ARibfCMhw
- If it had evolved, this organism had to have a kind of mutation first, a male or a woman ... It not is such a thing ... I am looking at it with certainty that you come from somewhere else.
- I wanted to do a chemical analysis of the sperm and the sperm in the womb a few days after it was placed .. what would happen if I took the thing and sowed it in the water?
- Is that embryo in the uterus an enzyme?
- I do not think you can develop as an organ when it is thrown into the water outside
- So the baby can not grow out in a place other than a mother's stomach, like an outside person.
- Can the first human be formed for this kind of water? .. mutation on mutation
-?

CURE

- Mother's milk
- If the first man is developing as male
- We can not talk about mother's milk.
- Otherwise,
- can not breed without semen
- They have to come out at the same time
- Women can produce milk.
- The reason for the formation of a mammal is that it can actually give milk.
- We can not have had such an original evolution!
-;)
- Do you realize you can produce milk, Noone?
- How does it feel?
- Do you think there are jinn?
- No comment?
- Hey Noone, 23 books were sold in Italy..I guess I will go there 2nd place in germany
- I need to learn Italian
- I need to read books in Italian.
- To there I have at least 10 artist friends and all of them painters
- I need 4 months calcination..
- Voglia a una donna bella

Noone:

-Translate, to all Italian

Artur:

- Yeah

Noone:

-Can be interesting

 - Intellectuals like us

-They look to us like aliens already..

Artur:

- Yes, unfortunately we are aliens, godless and perverted.

- I will go to Italy .. I want to write myself in Italian

Noone:

-Walk

- Salerno

- The venue of my choice

- I'il look at the language course.

Noone:

-No Italian

- But they all have an uncertainty, like the German-French mixture.

Artur:

- But they value the art.

- Especially poetry

Noone:

-Yes..

- That's the important thing..

Artur:

- a French singer medium celebrity

Noone:

-La comedia divina

Artur:

- Last year, he spoke of my poems.

- Est que son de jeuxqueste son des jeux
- I forget French.

Noone:

-I think that in Europe there is a British and a German
- Others were synthesized

Noone:

- It's called the Anglo-Germen,

Noone:

-I wanna live in London.
- 1 month is enough

Artur:

- London would be nice to you
- Live at Nothing Hill...
- Noone, actually, if you want to live in the UK, you'd better go to Edinburgh after a day of excitement, a wonderful city from the Middle Ages

Noone:

-Wanna go to the theater ,to watch Jude Law, Ralph Fienes

-Go out on the horse with the dogs

-Sit British hanging in a heavy gentlemen club..

-Go to opera

-Make Bouquet

-A little fog

-I want to hear the English talk to the cunts.

Artur:

- Scotland..

Noone:

CURE

-I do not want to live..

Artur:

- I recommend
- 1 month
- Edinburgh
- Full medieval

Noone:

-Can be..
- Super

Artur:

- I stayed 2-3 months there
- I know all about ..
- Super..

Noone:

-No country at the moment
- It does not interest me
- I mean another country

Artur:

- I went all over the UK
- Scotland I recommend you
- Structure of the city
- Old town is there
- Walk..
- English..
- It takes 3-4 days to understand.
- The money is also different.
- I wanted to go out with you ...
- https://youtu.be/MYfEBL1ItAE

- Listen to the opera.

- :) fuck opera..

- https://youtu.be/4JThPc33NJc

- This is for super friends like you

- Stay calm

- I am an artist who affixed the chart to all the UK

- Not in a gallery

- Read the lost philosopher

- I sent it to you

- :)

- Do you make if I ask you anything?

Noone: Yes i do, Artur ..

Artur:

- Get out of my life now!

Noone:

-What? Why Artur? Why are you doing this to me ?

- What have I done to you, Artur?

- Talk to me..

Artur:

- I think you're a scare Noone ... I've been calling you never answer the phone. 2 - 3 days later you never come back again .. You've read all the stuff I've written .. I've always tried to talk to you . but you preferred these texts..You did not do anything I wanted. You have been so excited by me many times that you have been so excited. But these excitements have always remained at that moment.It did not come back. I think that you can not do anything on your own by doing what you have to do. You have been blocked.Your final production capacity has fallen.

-You have been nothing but a robot for the last few months.

-I wrote you here to record everything that came to my mind.

Noone:

-Artur, what's wrong with you? Yes, you are right .. I made you very wrong .. I could not realize it at first what I did to you. I did not pay attention to it, I apologize .. Please forgive me ..

- Let's meet tomorrow with you Artur..What is it? I am so Sorry..

- Artur! Are you there?

Artur:

- I am here.Okay. Come to the place we met the first time ..

Noone:

-Okay .. I'll be there on time ..

Artur:

- Okay, I'il see you. I want to be alone now.

Noone:

- See you Artur ..

It was a silent story, it could have been a silent film. After that, the rumors, in the silence of abandonment, could never fit to that..

While Noone was sitting in one of those noisy cafes, waited to Artur quietly,and put her cigarette, her sunglasses and his lighter on the table.The broken sunlight was hitting her face and she wondered how to talk to Artur.It was a dialect for both of them.It was a love game that was only compressed by words, played by words.In fact, neither Noone nor Artur ever lived and could not live each other.Noone is immersed in thought,she started designing what Artur would say to the line.She thought it was very painful and she started to stir another cube of sugar.

- Artur, first of all I apologize to you very much. Forgive me, but I have been very honest with you and I have made a decision to tell you something. I want you to know that everything I tell you is true now. Maybe you can understand me better. I've been married before but I'm not. I have not felt like a married woman since my husband started cheating me with another woman for three years. I have not slept in the same bed with him for three years. I waited all the time, he did not turn back and still be with her.It is nice to for him come home and go on like it was nothing.This last passing time was really painful for me.I tried to divorce many times and it was not my strength.And you met me, we really did not live anything with you.Even we did not catch each other's eye .But what you wrote, what you told me, what you shared with me was very influential.I could not give an answer, my conscience did not allow this. I apologize to you very much.You filled that void in me.The pain of what you wrote to me was ointment for me. Now I understand how much I need you, how much you care about me, how you try to show me the meaning of life I can not understand. I am so sorry that I did it to you.I should have given more thought to you. I should have taken more care of you.While you are not a psychiatrist, you could notice the depression in myrself and you did heal myrself, you have come out and made me a perfect therapy and you saved me from depression. Without the need to use medication.However, I made you a patient treatment and diagnosed you every time ..I do not want to lose you, you are the man who illuminates my darkness, and I did not know your value.Do you forgive me? Let me make a new start with you, help me .. I do not want to resist anymore .. Will you start a new one with me?

Artur was not thinking about meeting Noone and would not go out to meet. He would have witnessed the unconscious love of two strangers who did not know each other. Artur noticed that Noone was in depression, and designed a virtual love in Noone's brain so that Noone could get out of this depression, allowing Noone to live this love life and get out of her depression.This was a new study for Artur and he developed a method that allowed his psychiatrist to get out of depression.The love was part of this cure and it worked. Noone ever thought about going into a much deeper depression after that.

Noone:
- Hello, Artur! Where are you ? I am waiting you ..
- Hello ... do you hear me?
- Artur !
- Talk to me ! Are you there ?

CURE

-Don't do that to me.

- Artur ...

DECISION

Artur:

-Sorry Noone, it's impossible for us to see you now, after I say these last things, I can not do things like that, to be with a woman married to a heir. It seems to me a very sick situation. I can now better understand why you have such severe depressions.It's impossible for you to know what I think right now. Now that everything you thought you'd expect me to be buried in that cave forever in a deep silence.Now I think it will be very beneficial to you.You can no longer know the value of the things in your hand and you can not resist happiness.I did not want to do this, but I did the right thing. Films also show the opposite why this is the case, but the end always ends up against the men. I'm doing the reverse. I am a person who has more self denial.For me, some pleasures do not really make a deep and exciting sense.Do not think this will force me.You may think that if you are to satisfy yourself like this. I hope that you do not try to get revenge for anything, the price may be even heavier for you. I do not need a ceremony for this thing.

Artur:
- Hello?
Sara:
- Hello ... Artur ..
Artur:
- Yes..
Sara:
-Hello, I'm Sara.
Artur:
-Sara?

Sara:

-Uff..You did not remember..We met at the Starbucks Cafe. You were looking for a seat to meet, and when you could not find it, you asked if you could sit down. I accepted it. We had a long chat and you gave me your phone.

Artur:

- Mmm. Yes, I remember, Sara.Whats up ?

Sara:

- I'm fine Artur, You did not call me for a long time.I am waited..Then decided to call..

Artur:

- Thank you, Sara, for thinking about me..Sorry.I was busy..

Sara:

- Where are you Artur now? What are you doing ?

Artur:

- I'm home, Sara. I do not do anything.

Sara:

- Come to me .. I'll have something to drink.

Artur:

- To you? Are you sure ?

Sara:

- Yes to me .. I'm sure ..

Artur:

- I do not know how?

Sara:

- It's better if you did not do anything right now, Artur.

Artur:

- All right, Sara. Where are you live ? Message me at the address ..

Sara:

- Okay Artur .. Come on .. I'm waiting ..

Artur:

- Okay I will come .

-Why did this come from? Sara..The bloody crazy people find me ..She is calling me the house without any hesitation.We do not even know each other..That is a reliable type.Life is a really talisman.Look at what you've been through and then look at what started ... I do not mind sometimes ... I'm sure I'm standing on a straight line.The sorrows ...The sorrows are intertwined with joy.Patience and delightful control.It's like protecting a person from major faults.It's always possible to talk about a divine justice. Let's see what you will tell Sara .What you've built in your mind for me ... we will see together ...

Sara:

- Aaa ... You're welcome, Artur.

- These flowers. Are these for me, Artur?

Artur:

- Yes, for you, Sara.

Sara:

- Thank you so much Artur..Come in ..

Artur:

- How big is your house, Sara.It is belong to you ?

Sara:

- Yeah Artur belongs to me.

Artur:

- You have a lot of Menora in your house .. Are you Jewish, Sara?

Sara:

- Yes, Artur ... How did you know of Menora?

Artur:

- I visited one of the nearby synagogues a few times.I like watching rituels..

- If you look at mythology, we are all Jews. Is not the first person Jewish ?

Sara:

-Yeah Artur .. I can not tell you I'm a very religious person.

- I do not know.

- There's wine.Let drink?

Artur:

- I do not drink, Sara. Please something without alcohol. I want coffee..

Sara:

- OK..

- Interesting .. I guess you are one of the rare men who rejected a woman's wine offer.

Artur:

- I suppose all the men you invite here agree to the wine offer, Sara.

Sara:

- What? I do not understand Artur ..

Artur:

- No sugar, for coffee Sara.

Sara:

- Ok...

Artur:

- You are one of the blondes with rare beauty in the city..I think so you have a lot of fans .. You are both rich and beautiful .. There must be many men who want to be with you .. Why did you call me? I'm the milk livered man..

Sara:

- Why are you talking like that, Artur?

Artur:

- I do not know.What think , i am talking..

Sara:

- Do you mind telling everybody, Artur?

Artur:

- I usually say ...

Sara:

- I got it.Coffee..

- Tell me what you're doing, Artur?

Artur:

- I do not do anything, Sara.

- What about you ?

Sara:

- I have a job we set up together with my husband on time, trying to keep it going.

Artur:

- I'm happy for you. Why did your husband die?

Sara:

- Suddenly got caught in pancreatic cancer and suffered in six months and passed away.

Artur:

- I'm so sorry for you. Rest in peace ..

Sara:

- Amen ...

- Is it heaven, Artur? Do you think there is something like that?

Artur:

- I do not know?

Sara:

- What are you saying ? God created Adam, and then he said to them, "There is a banned fruit here and there. Do not touch it." One day devil came to meet them who did not prostrate to Adam and tricked him for the banished fruit. They were all fired together from heaven. It must have brought a much more complex thing to God that created the world. Why did Satan have to prostrate to a man ? There was God. Weird .. and why God sent them together to World ? What a punishment.

Artur:

- Yes, it's strange Sara. Sometimes I think of them. I say ... that, The first human came to world really ignorant from heaven ? Some cosmic things come to mind.

People come to the world, these people have children. Are these brothers made first sex with each other? Brother sister? These strange brothers and sisters did kill each other. These people should be speaking a single language. After that, hundreds of languages are emerging. How is it? .What language did the first person speak? What language did people speak first in heaven? What was the first food to be eaten in the world? How did they discover sexual intercourse with each other? It does not take my mind ..questions..questions..

Sara:

- Where did we get here, Artur ..?

Artur:

- I believe you called me ..

Sara:

- Yes, I did.

Artur:

-Why did you call?

Sara:

- I liked you ...

Artur:

- But you do not like me, Sara.We can be friends

Sara:

- Is that so ?

Artur:

- It is.

- If you hope I'll sleep with you .. There will be nothing like this .. I do not like wine.

Sara:

- I did not expect anything like that. You are too bad man Artur..

Sara:

- Have you heard ?

Artur:

- Did I hear what?

Sara:

- Is there a sound from inside?

Artur:

- What sound ? I did not hear ..

Sara:

- I guess it's from the kitchen.

Artur:

- Let me take a look ... Sara ... There is nothing here and I have not heard any sound ...

- I have to go now, Sara. Thanks for the coffee.

Sara:

- No Artur stop..not go away .. do not leave me immediately ..

Artur:

- No, I will go ..

Sara:

- If you go ..i will kill myself, Artur.

Artur:

- What? Will you kill yourself? Are you okay, Sara?

Sara:

- I'm fine .. Do not go, Artur ..

- Do not leave me..

Artur:

- Sara, we just met.

- Sorry i have to go .see you again.

Sara:

- Yeah ? Really ?

Artur:

- I'm really will call you, Sara.

Sara:

- Promise ?

Artur:

- Come on ... I'm kissing you . Thank you for the invitation.

- What is this girl schizophrenic? All the folks find me .. What do I do? .. No, but there is a fear of abandonment in her. There is something else .. like a borderline .. she looks normal .. her conversations are organized ..She changed when I said I needed to go.She was completely different.Painful ..I am very sorry for her husband.Is it the traumas that has experienced after her husband death, turned into these episodes? Maybe I can help .. I can do what I can do .. I will do some more reviewing this .. I think I can solve with some hypnotic methods ..how will I persuade you? Maybe I could get a hypnosis by saying massaging. I need to have something to live with her to trust .She would like to go to bed several times.I can do it for a short time or a little.

- Now, let's look at the notes, and notice that the free associations are ruled in the brain. Kortex + substania nigra = stiratum> thalamus = internal clock process ..

So Talamus ... Broca's area from there ... What's going on here? Dopamin works here. If the brain could control the fake fiction and images that the voices brought to the venue here, this borderline person seemed to be able to heal .We will have to take a dopamine-balanced setting on her brain.

Artur:

- Hey, Sara. Are you in the mood?

Sara:

- I'm here Artur ...

Artur:

-What are you doing ? I was supposed to go to a really serious business meeting.

Sara:

- I'm at home Artur, I'm reading a book .. Not important ..

Artur:

- I want to give you a self-pardon. Can I come back to you today? Maybe I'll just try a new massage technique I first learned.

Sara:

- Do you know how to massage?

Artur:

- Yes, I have a few certificates.

Sara:

- It's interesting ... it's Artur.

Artur:

- You will definitely feel great. It will take 2 hours.

Sara:

- Thank you very much for coming back to me. I thought you would not call me again, you would not write me ..

Artur:

- No, my sweetheart.

-I had a hurray that day.

- I will come to your side soon.

Sara:

- OK, i am waiting ..

Artur:

- Hi, Sara,

Sara:

- Hi. Come in. What's this big bag?

Artur:

- Sara, its the massage table.

Sara:

- Ow.Too big

Artur:

-You know why it's so big ...You will see when i set it..

Sara:

- OK..

- Come back here, look what I'll show you ...

Artur:

- What are you going to show?

Sara:

- Come on.

- If i will keep your hands you do not be angry ...?

Artur:

- No..

Sara:

- Look, I did it last night after you left.

Artur:

- Woaw, are you a painter?

Sara:

- What do you think? I tried to tell you the anger that was in you in this mirror.

Artur:

- It's a great Expression.I liked.You are a surrealist..

Sara:

- Kiss me Artur ..

Artur:

- Shall I kiss ?

Sara:

- Kiss ...

Artur and Sara started kissing. Artur did not think about sleeping with Sara,While Sara was trying to strip him, Artur had already Hypnotized to Sara in a hurry after taking Sara's head in the palm of her hand and lightly touching it in the middle of her forehead.Artur put Sara in her bed first.He went inside and brought the massage table.He set the table in the bedroom and put Sara on the table.He went to the saloon again and moved the music set to the room.Now everything was ready.After installing the music set, he put on a CD that he could send isochronic messages to the brain.After passing by the tip of the head of the thigh and sending biomagnetic signals to Sara's brain by hand for 15 minutes.Sara's brain enabled her to scan itself.Process was started.We will see if he could get the right result.Sara had fallen into a deep sleep.An hour later Artur went to Sara's footsteps and sent some signals from there.Sara occasionally showed sudden reflex movements..It's a good sign.It may also have been noticed that Sara's skin became more vivid. Artur would be able to see the actual result two days after she woke up, and maybe he would have to do this a few more times.How he was going to tell Sara about it. He had to think about something.15 minutes before the end of the seance, he moved Sara to her bed again. Then he picked up the table and the music set, he returned to Sara. Slightly touching Sara's forehead, he woke her up.

Sara:

- What happened to Artur?

Artur:

- I guess you've had a blackout due to blood pressure. How do you feel now?

Sara:

- Actually, I feel great Artur .. Like being born again? How long time i sleeping here?

Artur:

- About two hours, Sara.

Sara:

- Have you been waiting for me for two hours?

Artur:

- Yeah..

Sara:

- You are a very good person. so glad i have you Artur. Artur ... I saw something in my dream while I was here. Artur ..

Artur:

- What did you see, Sara?

Sara:

- I saw my ex-husband, he threw his hand into the heart and took it out. It did not hurt at all. The heart was showing me the tips. I took it from his hand and put it back in. Then I woke up and saw you on my head.

Artur:

-You've had a different dream, Sara. You can make a picture about this dream.

Sara:

- Is not it ? Good idea ... you were going to have a massage.But could not..

Artur:

- Look at you, your face is laughing now.

- I will come back in a few days.Then i can make massage to you

Sara:

- Okay .. Many thanks, Artur ..

Artur:

- Now I'm going Sara, there are things I need to do ..

Sara:

- Okay Artur .. I'm send off you...

Artur:

- No, do not stand up, if you feel tired.

Sara:

- No Artur I feel very energetic, on the contrary .. I can start to do the painting that you mentioned after you go ..

Artur:

- Really ?

Sara:

- Yes, Artur. It might even be over when you come back.

Artur:

- Ok, then I'm going to wait for you to see the painting.

- See you .

Sara:

- See you ..

Artur:

- Waow.. its works..This time it did not show any reaction when I left the house. It seemed energetic as well as very calm and cool. After a few days, I can understand it more clearly. I have made a direct diagnosis .. Borderline ..! I have to take a few notes.

Borderline "personality disorder:

Here, in common with bipolar disorder, it is aimed to observe the effectiveness of mood stabilizers used in psychopharmacological treatment of "borderline" personality disorder (BPD). In this framework, we will attempt to observe the overlapping phenomenon of bipolar disorder with BPD and the characteristics of differential clinical diagnosis in the light of the literature.

Both disorders may exhibit common features in terms of diagnosis, overlap in phenomenological terms, and coexistence rates are also very high. In order for both disorders to be separated from one another, attention should be paid to the nature of mood swings, the type of impulsivity and the longitudinal course of disorders. Several studies have investigated the efficacy of mood stabilizers such as lithium, carbamazepine, oxcarbazepine, sodium valproate and lamotrigine in the management of BPD.

It is not easy to separate BPD from bipolar disorders. A very careful assessment is necessary. This distinction can also be beneficial from a treatment point of view. Numerous research results have been published on the efficacy of valproate and lamotrigine in the management of BPD. Findings related to other mood stabilizers are insufficient. The use of any medication in the treatment of BPD has not been endorsed by official authorities. Psychotherapeutic approaches are important in the treatment of BPD. However, a symptom-based approach has been proposed for the use of mood stabilizers.

BPD is defined as a continuous pattern that starts in young adulthood and emerges under various conditions, accompanied by significant impulsivity, which is inconsistent with the perception and emotion of the interpersonal relationships. Characteristically, Incessant perceptions of self-perception, impulsivity, repetitive behaviors related to suicide, fluctuation in affect, a constant sense of emptiness, intense anger, paranoid thought content, and sometimes severe dissociative symptoms may occur.

Since the BPD diagnosis has been included in the DSM classification, there is an intensive effort to include this disorder in I axis disorders.While some authors attempted to place a place in the schizophrenia spectrum of the BPD, more researchers tried to relate it to mood disorders.While priorities were associated with major depressive disorder, attention was then focused on bipolar disorder and this personality disorder was attempted to be located in the spectrum of bipolar disorders.Some researchers have suggested that the concept of bipolar disorder is used in a very narrow sense, in fact that this category of diagnosis covers a much wider area.These researchers have suggested that many cases of BPD are actually present in the spectrum of mood disorders and that correct identification and treatment can be done more effectively.

Akiskal's contribution to this debate has been more concrete and descriptive. According to Akiskal, BPD patients are those who have a clinical appearance that is continually shifting between depression and irritable hypomania, with a dimmer or less stable bipolar II disorder, and cyclothymic mimicry.In this case, they have to be involved in the bipolar spectrum and their treatment should be regulated. Akiskal suggested that histrionic, narcissistic and borderline personality disorders associated with depression should be included in the classification of " soft or bipolar disorders " (Soft bipolar disorders). Akiskal has sometimes suggested that these disorders progress to more severe (Type I and Type II) forms than more mild images of bipolar disorders.Akiskal tried to define the bipolar spectrum in a very wide range of diagnosis. According to this theory, the bipolar spectrum does not include only mania and hypomania, and includes the resulting cyclothymic and hyperthymic temperament.These two subtypes are also under the " insignificant

or light bipolar spectrum " dimension.The phases that begin in cyclothymic or hyperthymic temperament, puberty or early adulthood and are characterized by sudden transitions include only a few days of euthymic periods.Sometimes this is called the "ultra fast cycle". This definition is also typical of emotional fluctuations in borderline personality disorders. Therefore, Akiskal suggested that these cases should be evaluated in the bipolar spectrum. BPD is defined as a continuous pattern that starts in young adulthood and emerges under various conditions, accompanied by significant impulsivity, which is inconsistent with the perception and emotion of the interpersonal relationships.Characteristically, Incessant perceptions of self-perception, impulsivity, repetitive behaviors related to suicide, fluctuation in affect, a constant sense of emptiness, intense anger, paranoid thought content, and sometimes severe dissociative symptoms may occur.

Other authors have not accepted these views. In some cases they thought that these two disorders could be seen together, yet they thought that the BPD diagnosis constituted a separate diagnostic category and the classification in DSM was valid.

Several psychopharmacological agents have been tested for the symptoms of BPD patients. Among these, mood stabilizers have an important place. These drugs are mostly tested on impulse, anger, affective disorder, and depression. In some studies, such drugs have been found effective. In some studies the activities were disputed.

BPD and bipolar disorders are both severely severe and potentially potentially affecting various areas of life. Both disorders may exhibit common features in terms of diagnosis and may overlap phenotypically. Attention should be paid to the nature of the emotional episodes, the types of impulsivity and the longitudinal course of the disorders in order to be able to distinguish them. It is very important to make a correct diagnosis and to arrange treatment accordingly. It is not uncommon for both disorders to coexist and should not be overlooked.

According to the results of retrospective findings, it was found that accompanying BPD with bipolar disorder had no effect on clinical course, remission levels and hospitalization rates of functional status with respect to functional status. BPD accompanied by bipolar disorder is of greater importance in terms of the use of mood stabilizers in treatment. The coexistence of both disorders can increase the individual's self-directed violence.

There is more data available in the literature regarding the efficacy of valproate and lamotrigine. Other medicines are few.

Mood stabilizers have been approved by the Food and Drug Administration (FDA) for at least one of 3 phases of bipolar disorder (mania, bipolar depression, long term survival).

However, no drug, including mood stabilizers, has been approved by the FDA for the treatment of BPD. Only use of mood stabilizers in some symptoms is recommended. This suggests that the presence of BPD in the bipolar spectrum does not make much sense in terms of treatment.

Psychotherapeutic approaches, which can be regarded as psychosocial treatments, give hope in spite of the inadequate data on the treatment of CBF with mood stabilizers.

Psychotherapeutic approaches, which can be regarded as psychosocial treatments, give hope in spite of the inadequate data on the treatment of BPD with mood stabilizers. Among these approaches; Dialectical behavioral therapy, schema-focused therapy, and transfer-focused psychotherapies. As you can see, the efforts of the BPD to insist on placing bipolar disorders between places do not make a serious contribution to the treatment approach. Significant overlap of the diagnostic criteria in the DSM system does not mean that both disorder groups are exactly the same thing. However, it is a fact that it is not easy to distinguish bipolar disorders other than bipolar I disorder by BPD. Only inadequate decomposition efforts to be performed according to the diagnostic criteria in the DSM system are inadequate. It may also be beneficial from a treatment point of view to provide a more comprehensive assessment and resolution.

It is estimated that DBP is about 2% of the prevalence in general society. This ratio is about 1-2% in bipolar disorder. For bipolar spectrum distortions, there are also sources where this ratio is given as 5%.
In a comprehensive study of Paris and colleagues, it was emphasized that the incidence of bipolar I disorder in BPD patients was 5.6% and 16.1%. The average rate is around 9.2%. When bipolar II disorder is considered, this ratio is between 8% and 19%. The average rate is 10.7%. When two studies using structured diagnostic interviews with strong methodologies and having a sufficient sample size and based on 6 year longitudinal follow-up are examined, Bipolar disorder was detected at baseline in low-grade patients with BPD. Furthermore, these ratios were not different from the control groups. When another well-designed methodology was examined, bipolar I and II disorders were found at significantly higher rates in groups composed of BPD and other personality disorders (schizotypal, avoidant and obsessive-compulsive personality disorders). These ratios are 19.4% for BKB and 7.9% for the other group.

When the groups were followed longitudinally for 4 years; The incidence of bipolar I and II disorders was significantly higher in BMI group than other personality disorders. These ratios were found to be 8.2% and 3.1% respectively. Although these ratios show a moderately increased risk level in patients with BPD, major depressive disorder and substance abuse in BPD are considered to be very low in terms of risk ratios.

In studies investigating the rate of BPD in bipolar I disorder, very different results were found. These ratios vary from 0.5% to 30% and the average is 10.7%. However, these rates vary between 12% and 23% in bipolar II disorder, with an average of 16.6%. In a study that did not show a relationship between cyclothymia and BPD, the incidence of both disorders was found to be as high as 62%.

It is difficult to distinguish between bipolar disorder and BPD. Because in both disorders, patients exhibit affective irregularity, irritability and impulsivity. Maninin phenomenology is distinctly different from BPD. Factor analysis of manic symptoms distinguishes marked psychic and motor acceleration, psychosis and irritability. When factor analysis of BPD is performed, three characteristic factors are identified: impairment in interpersonal relationships, behavioral disorder or inconsistency, and affective disorder

In recent studies, several parameters were found to distinguish between the two disorders - the overlap.

These parameters are; The nature of the mood episodes, the type of impulsivity, and the length of the disorder.

Both disorders cause emotional variability and affective mobility. However, the phenomenology of mood episodes is different. The mood is characterized by wavy and negative affection in the BPD. This can be triggered by perceived stress factors or by stress factors resulting from interpersonal relationships. It is a transient nature that lasts from a few minutes to hours and is severely dependent on environmental factors. Mood swings in bipolar disorder are much longer and more spontaneous. Especially in bipolar disorder type I, there are much more prolonged periods of exuberance. In addition, affective variability in BPD is a characteristic aspect of emotional response. According to the information available, affective problems persist throughout life, even during childhood and even during infancy. However, there are interim periods in which there are no symptoms in bipolar disorder.

The sensory fluctuations in the BPD and bipolar II disorder are also differentiated by the types of emotions. Individuals who have been diagnosed with BPD show a fluctuation towards the rage, but the etiology is not frequent. In bipolar II, affective shifting is an euphoria or blistering. Slippage in the BPD is characterized by rejection or abandonment and is triggered by interpersonal stress factors. These conditions remain very problematic for the separation of BPD and fast cycle bipolar disorder from each other in bipolar disorders. While the duration of emotional episodes, qualitative emotional shift, recurrent triggering findings and elaborate assessment of longitudinal patterns are helpful in establishing a differential diagnosis between BPD and bipolar disorders, this does not prevent the continued difficulties in diagnosing fast cycling bipolar disorder forms.

Impulsivity is seen in both BPD and bipolar disorder. The distinctive feature of impulse is the unplanned motor impulsivity in the manic phase in bipolar disorder and the unplanned impulsiveness in the depressive phase. The unplanned impulsivity is also dominant in the BPD. The data support that the symptoms present in the BPD overlap more with the depressive pole of bipolar disorder.

Similarly, BPD can be distinguished by bipolar II disorder through the presence of hostility thoughts and the difference of impulse. Bipolar II disorder has an impulsiveness that is carefully related. This impulsivited attention can turn very quickly in another direction and is far from a goal. There is also an unplanned impulsiveness in the BPD. The highest impulsivity level in the population was found in individuals with BPD and bipolar II disorder. It was alleged that these individuals had behaviors that would harm them at a very high level. These findings have shown that, in appropriate situations, the diagnosis of both disorders can coexist. Clinically, impulsivity is believed to be more episodic in bipolar disorder than in BPD. However, situations such as substance abuse can make bipolar disorder more complicated; Impulsivity can also be seen in episodes during this period. Impulsive behaviors such as suicidal behaviors can be seen in both disorders, but bipolar disorder is usually seen in the depressive phase.

In BPD, it is generally associated with despair and is often the result of inability to overcome stress situations.

Traditionally, when the longitudinal trends of disorders are compared based on axis I and axis II, Mood disorders were thought to be cyclical and treatable, and it was thought that personality disorders persisted throughout life and were resistant to treatment. However, many studies have shown that bipolar disorder cases may also have a chronic headache, show long-lasting disease symptoms, and may prove symptomatic between episodes. However, in long-term follow-up studies, it has been determined that a significant proportion of individuals with BPD are no longer able to meet the criteria of impairment after many years. However, subclass core symptoms persist in the BPD. Even more dramatic impulsive and harmful behaviors resume, psychopathological findings continue in the field of affective and interpersonal relationships. However, incidents that do not involve partial remission can also be seen.

Psychotherapy remains central to the treatment of BPD. However, pharmacotherapy is also recommended in some cases. There is information that some drugs are effective in some symptom clusters and in crises. Among these medications, those used as mood stabilizers have an important place.

In a study involving 10 patients with a six-week, double-blind, placebo-controlled and BKB, lithium was compared with desipramine.

In this study, it was determined that lithium, especially BPD, has an effect on the basic psychopathological features of irritation, anger and self-harmful behaviors. In a surveillance trial conducted by Stein, it was reported that lithium and carbamazepine were effective on behavioral impairment and aggression in patients with BPD or antisocial personality disorder.

Gardner and Crowdry have shown that carbamazepine reduces the frequency and severity of uncontrolled behavior in studies involving 11 female patients. These results have been confirmed by other studies. One of them; 6-week, double-blind, controlled trial comparing carbamazepine (820 mg / day), alprazolam (4.7 mg / day), trifluoperazine (7.8 mg / day) and tranylcypromine (40 mg / day). Sixteen patients who had a cohort of hysteroid dysphoria with BPD were included in this study and the efficacy of carbamazepine was confirmed.

Controlled studies have shown that carbamazepine is good for not only impulsive aggression but also affective fluctuations. In a study by Denicoff et al., Which included 1257 individuals and included various neurological and psychiatric disorders, Carbamazepine, lithium, valproate, clonazepam, calcium channel blockers, phenytoin, antipsychotics and electroconvulsive therapy. In this study, carbamazepine was significantly superior to others in total healing scores in the subgroup with BPD diagnosis.

In a 12-week pilot study involving 13 patients with BPD who were followed up remotely; Statistically significant improvements were found in the anxiety, interpersonal relations, impulsivity, affective fluctuation and anger findings of the patients using oxcarbazepine.

Divalproex sodium is among the most widely studied mood stabilizers in patients with BPD. Wilcox has suggested that divalproex significantly reduces agitation in patients with BPD. In the group of patients with BPD and bipolar disorder, they found significant decreases in post-treatment agitation findings. These findings were confirmed by the researcher's later work using divalproex sodium.

Three placebo-controlled trials were then conducted. In a study conducted by Hollander and colleagues in which 16 patients with BPD were included in the study using double-blind and valproate (plasma level 80 g / ml); With significant improvements in global symptomatology, marked reductions in depressive symptoms, aggression, irritability, and suicidal ideation or behavior. In another double-blind study involving 52 consecutive 12-week, outpatient patients, the efficacy of valproate (average daily dose 1325 mg) on impulsive aggressiveness was confirmed. Frankmann and Zanari have found that valproate (plasma levels ranging from 50 to 100 g / mL) has significant effects on interpersonal sensitivity, anger, hostility and aggression in controlled 6-month studies involving 30 comorbid BPD patients with bipolar II.

The first use of lamotrigine in the treatment of BPD started with a study of Pinto and Akiskal. The study was open-ended, based on one-year follow-up and included 8 patients followed-up remotely. In this study, a significant improvement of 40% was detected in total functions. In addition, there have been reports of sexual impulsivity, substance abuse and significant improvements in suicidal behavior. In a review written by Green, it was reported that this drug, which is effective in mood disorders, is also effective in balancing mood in individuals who have received BPD.

Preston and colleagues found that 35 bipolar patients who retrospectively evaluated bipolar disorder in terms of BPD cohort received 40% of BPD. These patients have previously been evaluated for the efficacy of lamotrigine in two open-ended studies. The results showed that lamotrigine influenced all the characteristics of BPD and significantly improved impulsivity and mood swings.

In a more recent study, Tritt and colleagues found significant anger control improvements in patients treated with lamotrigine after 8 weeks in a study in which they included 24 female patients meeting the BPD criteria and compared lamotrigine with placebo.

Lamotrijin is a new group within the class of antiepileptics. It is structurally and pharmacologically unlike any other drug. It is thought to prevent kindling in cortex and amygdala. The anticonvulsive effect is thought to be through presynaptic neuronal membrane stabilization. Possible effect of lamotrigine is to inhibit excessive release of excitatory amino acids such as glutamate; It also blocks sodium channels and 5HT3 receptors. Although the antiepileptic effect is similar to phenytoin and carbamazepine, it is not chemically similar to these two anticonvulsives or other drugs. Side effects are less than carbamazepine, and it seems likely that future epilepsy will be selected as the first drug. One of the major difficulties in the treatment of psychotic disorders in epileptic patients is the risk of antipsychotic lowering the epilepsy threshold. It has been reported that the addition of lamotrigine to antipsychotics at low doses effectively treats the psychotic table as well as epilepsy. Lamotrigine has been used anticonvulsively in 1994 for FDA-approved 99 bipolar disorder that has been treated so far. In the largest study conducted, the treatment efficacy of lamotrigine was investigated and a moderate or marked improvement was noted in 68% of 41 depressive patients and 84% of 31 patients with hypomanic, manic or mixed hectare. A study involving Valproata lamotrigine has been ongoing from several days to about a year in good health. The use of lamotrigine 50-250 mg (mean 141 mg / day) in 16 treatment-resistant patients resulted in improvement in depressive symptoms in all patients, and only one patient had mixed hypomanic shifts in response to treatment.

Patients who did not respond were found to have one mixed depression and one depressed mania. In a study investigating the role of 5-HT1A receptors in the efficacy of lamotrigine, 10 healthy individualized 5-HT1A receptor agonists, ipsapiron, were administered to assess body temperature and plasma cortisol responses. Lamotrigine given as 100 mg daily for one week did not change the hypothermia or cortisol response. A small number of subjects and short-term studies thus failed to prove that 5-HT1A receptor function was involved in the mechanism of action of lamotrigine. Unlike other medications used in studies involving mood disorders, it is suggested that lamotrigine be used for depression of bipolar disorder rather than antimanic and protective treatment. Lamotrijin's rapid effect is a feature that has been shared by many physicians working in the field of mood disorder but has not yet been established with controlled studies to date. In many congresses, symposiums, etc., it is stated that Lamotrigine is remarkably effective within 1 week from the day of application of BP disease in the depressive phase. Meanwhile, besides the various side effects, it has been reported that the most common side effect is rash (5-10%), which is also associated with rapid dose escalation. My clinical observations confirm this. The most serious side effect reported is Stevens-Johnson Syndrome.

- Another issue that comes to mind is mood disorder and epilepsy relationship:

Mood disorders are an important psychiatric comorbidity affecting the quality of life and prognosis of epilepsy. The relationship between depression and epilepsy is bi-directional. The risk of developing depression among epileptic events is higher than that of healthy controls, and the risk of developing epilepsy among depressive episodes is higher than that of healthy controls. Succinct epilepsy five times, temporal lobe epilepsis 25 times more. The independent risk of suicide in epilepsy depression increases even more in the presence of depression. The common pathway between epilepsy, depression and suicide is hypofrontality and irregularities in serotonin metabolism.

While the index provides more information about depression, bipolar disorder

Related data is more limited. However, emotional disorder is more frequent than it is thought to be mania and mixed periods characterized by irritability. Both disorders are cyclic and may become prolonged. Irregularities in the firing phenomenon, neurotransmitter, voltage-gated ion channels and secondary messenger systems are the alterations introduced in the etiology of both disorders. Emotion

Anticonvulsant drugs with regulatory effects are the common treatment point.

Understanding the mechanisms of action of these drugs will shed light on pathophysiological processes. In this article, the relationship between epilepsy and mood disorders, comorbidity, secondary conditions and treatment options in both cases are discussed.

Mood disorders (MD) are an important psychiatric comorbidity affecting the quality of life and prognosis of epilepsy. The relationship between depression and epilepsy has been discussed by both Hippocrates and Areteus in ancient times. Griesinger in the 1850s and Robertson melancholy in the 1900s

And depression. The relationship between depression and epilepsy is bi-directional. The risk of developing depression among epileptic events is higher than that of healthy controls, and the risk of developing epilepsy among depressive episodes is higher than that of healthy controls. Succinct epilepsy five times, temporal lobe epilepsis 25 times more. Epilepside depression

The independent risk of suicide is further increased in the presence of depression. The common pathway between epilepsy, depression, and suicide is hypofrontality and serotonin metabolism

Irregularity.

While the index provides more information about depression, bipolar disorder is more limited, particularly in the national diet. However, emotional disorder is more frequent than it is thought to be mania and mixed periods characterized by irritability. Bipolar disorder and epilepsy share some common features.

The kindling phenomenon, described in 1960, is conceptualized as spontaneous paroxysmal activity induced by precursor brain stimulation. Similar mechanism is most common for psychiatric disorders, including bipolar disorder

. The anticonvulsive efficacy of electroconvulsive therapy (ECT) with the effect of enhancing the seizure threshold is based on the assumption that it is a suprarenal stimulus and will not cause the kindling mechanism. Epilepsy and bipolar disorder are both cyclic and prolonged. Ignition phenomenia, neurotransmitter irregularities, irregularities in voltage-gated ion channels and irregularities in secondary messenger systems are the changes suggested in the etiology of both disorders. G proteins, phosphatidylinositol,

Proteininase C, domain-rich C kinase substrates, and changes in calcium activity. [1] The common mechanism in the ion channels is the antiepileptic effects of regulating the potassium output and the calcification antagonistic anticindling effects. Anticonvulsant drugs with mood stabilizing effects are the common treatment point. Understanding the mechanisms of action of these drugs will shed light on pathophysiological processes.

The aim here is not to look at the relationship between epilepsy and mood disorders, comorbidity, secondary conditions, and treatment options in both cases. For this purpose, I summarize the results of the study on the effects of variable phenomenological phenomena and anticonvulsants in the subheadings of depression, suicide and bipolar spectrum disorders.

Prolonged depressive mood has been reported in status epilepticus, petit mal status, temporal lobe status, nonconvulsive status and partial status epilepticus.

This condition was accepted as a secondary picture for organic brain disease and the treatment of ictal activity with anticonvulsant drugs

Has been proposed. On the other hand, it is emphasized that depressive mood around seizures may have serious consequences such as suicide. Periactal depression is not very common and there are not many publications about it. Interictal depression is the most common and clinically important situation among epileptic individuals. Moderate and severe depression in 20% of temporal epilepsy patients, 62% of patients with complex partial seizures, and 38% of depressive episodes present at life time.

Depression scores in temporal lobe epilepsy (TLE) are higher than in generalized (generalized) seizures. Indaco reports that at least 50% of all epileptic events meet the criteria for depression according to DSM-III-R. Mendez interictal depression is a frequent and unusual reaction to healthy controls in epileptic individuals, As a range extending.

Signs of clinical appearance of interictal depression; Anxiety, neuroticism, hostility, obsessions, addiction, change in sex, paranoia, irritability, lack of humor, absurd affection and

They are. In a study investigating whether some personality traits affect mood phenology, there was a difference in personality traits between the 5-Dimensional Personality Inventory (NEO-PR) and the Minessa Multidimensional Personality Inventory (MMPI-2) in 23 right, 21 left, and 24 temporal lobe out.

Psychotic symptoms may be seen in interictal depression. There were 66 cases of sera and 53 cases of psychotic symptoms (mood and incongruent delusions and hallucinations).

The drug is not more than an epileptic depressive event in the interictal depression, as it is thought to be overdose and self-injurious behavior. It has been shown that the severity of attack is also related to the duration of epilepsy. While the presence of depression and attempted suicide in family narratives was found high by some researchers, this finding was not confirmed elsewhere. Interictal depression is usually a non-endogenous, moderate-severe depressive disorder. Whether or not there is a bioelectric projection of depression is often asked. Different types of antidepressants used in the treatment of depression affect the seizure threshold differently. Auditory, visual and somatic stimuli provide specific and sex-specific findings for epilepsy, schizophrenia, bipolar disorder and healthy control groups. In a study comparing 16 episodes of major depression with 16 episodes of organic brain dysfunction or organic brain dysfunction, epileptiform activity was not found significantly in the first group with a large number of unusual features. High temporal delta amplitudes and interhemispheric temporal delta asymmetry epilepsy and organic brain dysfunction Have been found more frequently. However, the point of whether electroencephalographic (EEG) changes are a product of antidepressant treatment is open to debate. When pilocarpine is administered to lithium-administered rats, these animals experience a seizure and this seizure is defined as a limbic seizure syndrome.

Just as rats with high levels of brain inositol do not exhibit this seizure syndrome, this picture can be reversed with myoinzitol. It should be remembered that lithium at this point reduces brain inositol. Destroyed mice with inositol monophosphatase 1 and sodium myoinositol transporter 1 genes undergo seizures with pilocarpine as if lithium had been given. Pilocarpine susceptibility, in other words animals with inositol deficiency, are prolonged inactivity dur- ing challenging swimming testing. This is synonymous with depressive effect. From here, the inositol deficiency is matched to the lithium-like effect. The fact that seizures are not a component of bipolar disorder is neglected, although it is also suggested as a projection of mania therapy in model animal studies. In another study, anhedonia and hopelessness-like behaviors, which occurred in rats with lithiumchloride and pilocarpine status epilepticus, developed spontaneous repetitive seizures were considered as a model of depression and a disorder in the hypothalamopituitary adrenal (HPA) axes of these animals and in the serotonergic communication between the raphe and the hippocampus. State and depression, 20 mg / kg / day fluoxetine was given for 10 days, and in the forced swimming test, immobilization time was shortened and inhibition was observed in the cycle of serotonin in the hippocampus.

Tough swimming test performance does not improve when there is a reduction rather than an inhibition. Behavioral equivalence of depression and antidepressant resistance support this hypothesis that other mechanisms besides the serotonergic pathway are needed.

Some studies have suggested a relationship between mood and antiepileptics, some of which have not been validated for some time. This has been first suggested by Emrick in 1974 for Dolby in 1981 and Post for valproate (VPA) in 1984 for carbamazepine (CBZ) with positive psychotropic effects of anticonvulsants . In the same years, there have been reports of phenobarbital depression, suicidal thoughts and behavioral adverse effects. In the meantime, vigabatrinin has been shown to be an agent supporting mood. The new lamotrigine is compared with placebo, with a positive psychotropic effect on feelings of wellbeing, functionality and quality of life in addition to seizure control Lt; / RTI & gt; In an open study with levatiracetam, a 31% remission rate was reported in bipolar depression, but it has been suggested to support this finding with placebo-controlled studies. Biofeedback and relaxation techniques are effective in seizure control as well as depression in epilepsy cases. Psychotherapy is very important in the depression of these cases, especially in terms of the psychosocial causes of mood changes and the processing of stigmatization. Supportive therapy is suggested alone or with structured therapies (cognitive-behavioral therapy or interpersonal therapy). Psychotherapy is more effective with the use of antidepressants.

In a retrospective study of 19 antipsychotic drug candidates in epilepsy patients, 161 mg / day doxepin was reported to reduce both seizure frequency and depression scores. In a double-blind placebo-controlled study with Robertson and Trimble, 42 patients were compared with amitriptyline and nomifen They found that nomifensin was more effective on depression scores at 12 weeks. It should not be forgotten that the antidepressants (amoxapine, bupropion, clomipramine, maprotiline, mianserin, trazodone) except the whole monoamine oxidase inhibitor (MAOI) lowered the seizure threshold in the same study. MAOI and selective serotonin reuptake inhibitors (SSRIs) are more safe. In these cases, moclobemide may be a good option for removing psychomotor and cognitive impairment and sedative effects of anticonvulsants. It should not be forgotten that antidepressant withdrawal syndrome may increase the number of seizures during epileptic events. There is also a risk of status epilepticus. In addition, antidepressants can also affect the blood level of antiepileptics. For example; Imipramine and notriptyline increase the phenytoin activity. Carbamazepine toxicity may develop with biloxazin. SSRIs are a safe choice as opposed to the risk of suicide and suicide attempts in epileptic patients. Electroconvulsive therapy (ECT) stands as an option when lethargy and paranoid agitation become a risk. Paradoxically, the seizure threshold may increase during these events. There is also an anticonvulsive activity of ECT with the effect of boosting the seizure threshold. The kindling phenomenon, described in 1960, is conceptualized as spontaneous paroxysmal activity induced by precursor brain stimulation. It has been suggested that similar mechanisms may be applicable to many psychiatric disorders, including mood disorders. On the other hand, ECT is supposed to be a suprathreshold stimulus, presumably not causing kindling, but there are doubts about it. Bitemporal ECT application was found to be faster and more effective when compared to bifrontal and right unilateral electrode applications.

Epilepsy and bipolar disorder share some common features, and a number of studies have been carried out that address many of the features of this association and treatment approaches. The most important of these features is the cyclicality and continuity of both. Ignition phenomenia, neurotransmitter irregularities, irregularities in voltage-gated ion channels and irregularities in secondary messenger systems are the changes suggested in the etiology of both disorders. G proteins, phosphatidylinositol, proteinkinase C, domain rich C kinase substrates, and changes in calcium activity. The common mechanism in the ion channels is the antiepileptic effects of regulating the potassium output and the calcification antagonistic anticindling effects. Anticonvulsant drugs with mood stabilizing effects constitute the common treatment point, which will shed light on the pathophysiological processes of understanding the mechanisms of action.

We do not have standards for how treatment should or should be done when epilepsy and bipolar disorder coexist. The information available for this situation reflects the practice that exists in clinical practice. Ishihara and colleagues found that mood disturbance was more frequent among carbamazepine users in 44557 epileptic patients in 1997-2007, while gabapentin and clonazepam were the most commonly prescribed drugs in these types of episodes. Bipolar disorder was found in patients with comorbid epilepsy monotherapy as carbamazepine, valproate , Lamotrigine and oxcarbazepine can be used. On the other hand, in an open-label study involving 42 drug trials and 11 different agents, these drugs were found to be successful in 30 out of 38 patients. It has been reported that 7 cases of serous lithium in 8 cases have bipolar disorder without worsening of seizures and 1 case of both cases have corrected it. Cognitive functions of anticonvulsants The effect on the bipolar disorder alone is considered important. In one study, the effects of antiepileptic drugs and lithium on cognitive functions (memory, attention, reaction time, speech rate, psychomotor speed) were investigated with 159 bipolar disorder and lamotrigine, oxcarbazepine, lithium and topiramate were found to be the least deteriorating agents. It has been shown that carbamazepine has more negative effects on cognitive function. The effect of anticonvulsants on cognitive functions will become even more important when epilepsy and bipolar disorder are involved. Carbamazepine, oxcarbazepine and valproate are agents that use intracellular pathways. They also use lamotrigine, gabapentin, and pregabalin voltage-gated Na and Ca channels. Topiramate, gabapentin, tiagabin and levatiracetam, which increase GABAergic conduction and decrease glutamatergic. These agents, which use the third mechanism, may have an anxiolytic effect, but the mood stabilizing effects are limited. In an open study conducted with levatiracetam, although 31% of cases with bipolar depression are reported to be improved, this disease should be supported with placebo-controlled studies. Antipylactic drugs, especially carbamazepine and valproate, which are predominant in sedative effect, have antimanic, anxiolytic and hypnotic effects. At the same time, however, they also have fatigue, disturbance of attentiveness and depression. It is known that the active anti-epileptic medications, especially felbamate and lamotrigine, increase attention and have antidepressant properties. However, the anxiety of these drugs, Kesebir et al. Current Approaches to Psychiatry Psychiatry also has agitation and insomnia features. These features should be considered and cared for in treatment.

Mood swings and irritability are more common than suspected mixed episodes and mania epileptic events.The rate of epileptic pure bipolar disorder is 1.4%. When included in the phenotypic variant, intericard dysphoric disorder, preiscal dysphoria and postictal hypomania or mania, this rate is 11.8%. The incidence of epileptic pure bipolar disorder is 1.4% A rise. The acute unstabilized depressive syndrome, which differs from depressive, rapid onset, and ending with interictal dysphoric disorder with psychomotor agitation and relatively low insight, expands this field. The most important reflection of this situation is that these cases do not respond well to the antidepressant. In addition to their prevalence, not only depression, but also hypomania and mania, also deteriorate the quality of life when epileptic events occur independently of education, work, substance use disorders and other comorbidities. The effect of anticonvulsant drugs on cognitive function is considered as the only bipolar disorder. Epilepsy and bipolar disorder will become even more important when they are involved. On the other hand, anticonvulsant drugs have depressant (negative psychotropic) and enhancer (positive psychotropic) effects. In the presence of concomitant mood disorder, appropriate treatment choices must be made in both situations. Physicians dealing with epilepsy should be more aware of the symptoms of the broad and complex bipolar disorder spectrum, inform their patients and relatives about it, and implement comprehensive treatment interventions.

- Now I see how right I am. The method I used to correct these extreme abstractions needed placebo attachment. I'm doing this using magnetic energy.

- I will decide whether to hypnotize her again in the second meeting with Sara.

Sara:
- Hey, Artur. Are you in the mood?
Artur:
- I'm here, Sara.
Sara.
- What are you doing ? Come to me tonight ..

Artur:

- I'm working ... It's fine.

Sara:

- We can eat pizza.

Artur:

- I have not eaten a pizza in a long time, Sara.

Sara:

- Okay, I'll get you a nice pizza.

Artur:

- I will be there at 7 .

- See you ...

Artur:

- Hi, Sara.

Sara.

- Hello, Artur ... Come on in. Massage table again ?.

Artur:

- Yes, it was last time ...

Sara:

- Come on, dinner's ready.

Artur:

- They look great.

Sara:

- Let's get started Artur ... Tell me, who did you live with?

Artur:

- Alone..

Sara:
- Who's cooking you?

Artur:
- Me ...

Sara:
- Is not it so difficult?

Artur:
- No, Sara, I'm so happy.

Sara:
- Do not you wanna come and live here with me?

Artur:
- I do not know, I guess No ..

Sara:
- I understand.

- Do you want to watch a movie with me? I found a different film.

Artur:
- Ok ..What is name of film ?

Sara:
- ' By the Sea '

Artur:
- Who's playing ?

Sara:
- Brad Pitt and Angelina Jolie.

- It's a quiet movie.We can rest..

Artur:
- Ok ..I will.

- 'I see an awesome normalization in this girl.Let's see that you succeeded Artur. Watch the film and go on and on your way ..'

- It's a great love movie. They did very good psycho-analysis.
Sara:
- Yes, Artur, I liked too much...Stay here tonight.
Artur:
- I can not do it, Sara, I have to go.I am very sorry to have to stay up early in the morning.
Sara:
- What are you going to do, Artur?
Artur:
- I have a job interview, it's important to me.
Sara:
- You can get out of here.
Artur:
- Thanks I would love to stay with you, but in the morning I will have to prepare something at home.
Sara:
-You know, I will not argue.
Artur:
-Thanks for your understanding ..
Sara:
- I thank you for coming.

Artur:

- I could not massage again ... but already I saw you so relaxed anymore ...

Sara:

- Yes, I feel so great, I do not need to take a break.Maybe another day.

Artur:

- When do you want to ...

- Okay ... I have to go right now.

Sara:

- Sure.

Artur:

- See you again ,Sara..

Six weeks later ...

Sara:

- Hey Artur ... Are you there?

Artur:

- I am here .

Sara:

- How are you ? What are you doing ?

Artur:

- I'm in the abroad, Sara ..

Sara:

- It is.Really?

- I have a good news for you.

Artur:

- What is it?

Sara:

- This is spring, so I'm marrying in two months.

Artur:

- Wow, what happened?

Sara:

- After you, I started to talk with my first love from high school. He was married, he had ended his long marriage. We started to see him again and we decided to got married.

Artur:

- I'm very happy with this news Sara .. I wish you happiness ..

Sara:

- We are married on March 27th. I'd like to invite you, too.

Artur:

- I would love to come, Sara, but I will be abroad for a long time.

Sara:

- Okay, whatever you want ..

Artur:

- But please tell me where the marriage ceremony will be.

- Even if I can not come, I want to send you something.

Sara:

CURE

- Thank you Artur ..so glad i have you ..

Artur:

- I thank you for the invitation.

- See you ...

Sara:

- See you..

- Artur ...!

- Sorry ...

- Thank you so much ....

-The End-

www.ingramcontent.com/pod-product-compliance
Lightning Source LLC
Chambersburg PA
CBHW030608220526
45463CB00004B/1216